Communication in Nursing Practice

Communication

Eleanor C. Hein, R.N., M.S.

Associate Professor
School of Nursing
University of San Francisco

in Nursing

Practice

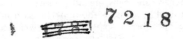 7218

LITTLE, BROWN AND COMPANY • BOSTON

Library of Congress catalog card No. 73-1420

ISBN 0-316-35448

Printed in the United States of America

With each passing year, my mother has made life fuller, more enduring, and infinitely precious. This book is for her, with love.

Contents

Preface

THERE IS NO "BEST" METHOD of communicating effectively with patients. The various patients whom we encounter have diverse backgrounds and outlooks on the world and its events, which preclude any hope we may have to confine them to some predetermined category. Similarly, we meet our patients with communication styles uniquely our own, formed in the past and crystallized in the present.

With our first encounters with patients, we begin a lifetime of repeated attempts to *use* variety to *meet* variety — the variety of communication approaches and styles that can influence our patients toward constructive decisions and insights about the level and quality of their health and health care. Central to this variety is the routing system that leads each nurse through the components of the communication process.

Communication in Nursing Practice is designed to take the reader along the route, and points out various communication skills, areas of knowledge, attitudes, and sociocultural influences essential to any concerned and purposeful approach taken to communicate effectively with patients.

The use of such a routing system in examining the process of communication may help diminish the myth that communication is too abstract a concept to learn. The more communication approaches we have, the more we will try; the more experience we gain through them, the more knowledgeable and helpful we will become; and the more varied the approaches we employ in professional nursing practice, the more we convey to each patient what he may rightfully expect to receive — individualized nursing care.

Eleanor C. Hein

Acknowledgments

IN EXPRESSING GRATITUDE to those people who have invested devotion, minds, and hearts in the creation of this book, words seem far too inadequate. There are never enough words to convey what their support, encouragement, and faith in me have meant. These few, perhaps, may serve as a beginning.

No effort of value (and writing is no exception) can grow in an atmosphere that stifles its accomplishment. Actualization of an effort occurs when it is allowed to thrive in the richness and receptivity of ideas, where its growth is nurtured with hope, and where, during moments of uncertainty, it is nudged along with unceasing confidence and enthusiasm.

Such an atmosphere is possible only if the people in it make it so. I am fortunate indeed to work with the people on the nursing faculty of the University of San Francisco. I would like to express particular appreciation to Sr. Mary Geraldine McDonnell, Dean of the School of Nursing, for her unfailing faith in my efforts and for her generous encouragement.

To the many students whom I have met in the mutual experience of learning, I extend a very special acknowledgment. It has been a pleasure to see them grow in their understanding and in their compassion for others. The ideas they have shared, the questions they have posed, the problems they have tried to solve, and the many patients they have cared for and about have served as sources of inspiration. All their experiences have added immeasurably to the development and, I hope, to the usefulness of this book.

I especially wish to thank Mrs. Ruth A. Wiens, Assistant Dean, University of Oregon School of Nursing, who read earlier versions of my manuscript. Her

xii ACKNOWLEDGMENTS

many helpful suggestions contributed much to the improvement of this book.
She assisted in other very special ways too numerous to list here, but for which
I thank her most sincerely. My thanks also to Miss Helen Robillard, who read
various sections of my manuscript and offered many pertinent and useful
comments.

Finally, searching paragraphs for a split infinitive or a dangling participle
were wise editors ready with advice, encouragement, and sharp pencils to help
me say what I wanted to say. My sincere gratitude to Mrs. Joan McClure
Guziec, who filled that capacity so well throughout the preparation of this
book, and to Mr. Robert M. Davis and Mrs. Deanna St. Aubin, who, as manuscript editors, thoughtfully supervised its final stages.

To each and all, my grateful thanks.

E. C. H.

Human language is like a cracked
kettle on which we beat out tunes for
bears to dance to, when all the time
we are longing to move the stars to pity.

— Flaubert

One must learn by doing the thing;
for though you think you know it
you have no certainty, until you try.

— Sophocles

1

The Communication Model

The Use of Models in Nursing

OF ALL THE EXPLOSIONS that have taken place in the past twenty years, the knowledge explosion has hurled more bits and pieces of information than we ever dreamed possible. Communication media and skills represent only a fragment of this phenomenon, but in nursing, such skills have become one of the major tools used to make nursing theories, concepts, and principles a reality in professional practice.

The study of communication skills is to most people an intellectual abstraction, especially to students entering nursing. They think that talking with people in need is just something you do, something that just comes. That one must relearn to communicate is an insult to them, because it is an ability they feel they already possess, and justifiably so. The abstraction is not looked upon favorably by students, who are impatient to become more involved with patient activities in nursing — the doing and the dramatics of what they feel constitutes real nursing with real (i.e., sick) patients.

All of us utilize our communication skills *as if* we were operating on some plan or design. The reason for the abstraction often is that we are not *aware* of the plan before, during, or even after we have completed the communication. If a verbal exchange results in a favorable response, we often think we have been lucky. This questionable conclusion promotes frustration, particularly when we are asked to be more specific about what we really do when we communicate with each other.

MODELS: THEIR CONSTRUCTION

One method of looking at the way we communicate is by plotting the process. This can be done by constructing a model, through which we scale down a broad concept such as communication into workable components.

Models can give structure and substance to a concept that previously had none, and they give clarity to situations in which ambiguity left us confused. They also help us to see the elements involved in the process and to explain or predict the sequence of events so that we need not rely on our intuition or trust our luck.

Models can be constructed for any sequence of events, which follow a step-by-step progression in which each step is dependent upon the one preceding it. When the sequence has been completed, the outcome is successfully accomplished. If the outcome is incorrect, the sequence must be retraced until the error is located and corrected.

Our body functions involve a variety of sequential events, including the circulatory, nervous, lymph, and digestive systems. Our circulatory system, for example, is dependent on the sequence that involves the elasticity and patency of blood vessels, the aeration of blood, and the pulsating rhythm of the valves and chambers of the heart. When these events occur within the circulatory system in an orderly and precise way, the outcome is a healthy, functioning body. When the sequence is disrupted by a clot or an irregular heartbeat, our ability to function is impaired. In order to regain our health and our ability to function, the circulatory system must be examined and the error (i.e., symptom) located and corrected.

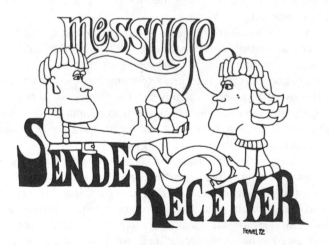

Fig. 1. Visual representation of a communication model.

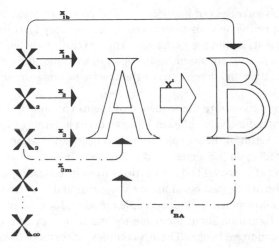

Fig. 2. In this complex communication model, the communicator (A) selects and condenses the stimuli in his sensory field and transmits its message (X^1) to B, who may or may not have all or part of the same stimuli in his own perceptual field (X_{1b}). Intentionally or not, B transmits feedback (f_{BA}) to A. (From B. H. Westley and M. S. MacLean, Jr. *Journalism Quarterly*, 34:34, 1957.)

Similarly, sequential events occur in other daily activities. The billing procedure in a department store is an example. If there has been an incorrect billing, the credit department must locate the error within the procedure. The sequence involved in placing a long-distance call, as another example, must be orderly for the call to be completed. At times it is possible to hear parts of this sequence while waiting for the phone to ring and a voice to answer. A busy signal indicates that the sequence of events leading to the completion of the call has been interrupted, and the call cannot be completed unless the sequence is begun again by redialing the phone number.

The sequence of events concerned with the arrangement and dissemination of information through the medium of a telephone call prompted scientists of the telephone industry to transcribe it into a visual model. Early ones were composed of a sender, a receiver, and a message. (See Figure 1.) As time passed, more complex models were devised to explore communication phenomena. (See Figure 2.)

MODELS: THEIR PURPOSE

The concrete substance provided by a conceptual model makes the abstraction of communication less overwhelming. A model provides form and utility, through which nursing knowledge can be integrated because it helps us to observe, predict, and understand what has taken place when two people have communicated.

Use of models increases our knowledge about communication skills, but they should not be the only instruments used because they can oversimplify and distort elements within the exchange. Their exclusive use limits the choices (e.g., various theories of communication) open to us in the study of interpersonal communication and deprives us of the diverse information the field can offer.

As these explorations into the sequence of events continued, other industries began to understand the value of examining an event in terms of its sequential properties. The result of these explorations has been automation. It has assisted industry by speeding up the sequence of events, which in turn has increased productivity and efficiency. The implications from investigating sequential events within the health sciences alone are staggering and have only begun to be explored. The development of more complex models, for example, has provided us with more information about the sequence and frequency of events within a given communication exchange. Though complex, these models have reiterated what previously had been a hope: that explanation and prediction *are* possible if a given communication sequence is examined with care.

A COMMUNICATION MODEL

We have said that models give substance to a concept in addition to having form and utility of their own. In Figure 3 the model is comprised of six elements:

1. The referent
2. The source-encoder
3. The message
4. The channel
5. The receiver-decoder
6. Feedback

Every encounter we have with another person, whether spontaneous or deliberate, begins with an idea — a reason for engaging in a verbal exchange. Often we are not aware of the reason; nevertheless, we operate *as if* it were preplanned. There are many interpersonal encounters in which we are aware of a reason. Wanting to ask parents for an increase of allowance or to ask an instructor for a time extension for an assignment activates the need for a communication contact. Our model must begin with that idea, that *referent*. A referent is "a wide range of objects, acts, situations, idea or experiences" [1]. Any one of these items or a combination of them prompts the source-encoder to initiate action in order to convey the message contained in the referent.

The source-encoder is a term that describes one person who talks with another. Our ability to form, use, and understand the messages we transmit is continually influenced by numerous factors, which David Berlo considers to include our communication skills, our attitudes, our levels of knowledge, and

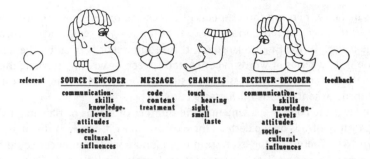

referent	SOURCE - ENCODER	MESSAGE	CHANNELS	RECEIVER - DECODER	feedback
	communication- skills knowledge- levels attitudes socio- cultural- influences	code content treatment	touch hearing sight smell taste	communication- skills knowledge- levels attitudes socio- cultural- influences	

Fig. 3. A basic communication model. (The illustration, drawn for this book, was adapted from the following sources: the portion based on Berlo's SMCR Model was from *The Process of Communication* by David K. Berlo, copyright © 1960 by Holt, Rinehart and Winston, Inc., used by permission of Holt, Rinehart and Winston; the remainder from *Speech Communication: A Behavioral Approach* by Gerald R. Miller, p. 73, copyright © 1966, by The Bobbs-Merril Company, Inc., used by permission of the publisher.)

our sociocultural system [2]. These factors are never static; indeed, they are always changing, always being modified as we change and are modified by the events that surround us. Whenever we interact in the role of the source-encoder we must consider these influences in order to understand not only our own communication, but also the communicative behavior of others.

Our ability to absorb the experiences we encounter is limited if we do not possess the ability to encode them into a form recognizable by others. The vocal mechanisms used in speech, the motor skills used in writing, and the language peculiar to a specific culture are encoding skills possessed to some degree by every human being. Similarly, the use of gestures and other non-verbal behaviors is an encoding ability, which often bridges the verbal gaps encountered by people who speak different languages.

The ideas and experiences we have as the source-encoder are, at this stage, still intangible. To make them come alive we must change that intangible invention into "an actual physical product," which in the communication model is labeled the *message* [3]. Regardless of the physical product — be it a sketch, a letter, or a conversation with a close friend — it remains our message, the concrete expression of our ideas and our experiences.

All of us are aware that a message does not just appear. Think about it! Messages, like communication in general, are not a matter of luck. Every day we deliver messages of varying kinds and lengths *as if* we actually knew what operations were involved. Of course, not all of us convey our thoughts with the adroitness of a Noel Coward or with the eloquence and cadence of a Winston Churchill. Still, we do possess certain verbal agilities and abilities unique to our individual communication style.

It follows, then, that if our message is understood, we must be doing something right, but the obvious facts are often the first to be overlooked.

In this instance there are three aspects of a message to consider. In order to convey a message, we must arrange it so that it has some semblance of recognizable order. In the English language, this requirement is filled by the sentence because it is "a series of words in connected speech or writing, forming the grammatically complete expression of a single thought" [4]. The order established through sentences is the *message code* [5].

Whatever the code is — a sentence, the number of sharps or flats in music, or the variety of oils on a palette — the expression of it becomes the *message content* [6]. Therefore, the expression from a number of sentences could be a book, from sharps and flats a symphony, or from the mixture of oils a landscape or portrait. Finally, no message can be sent unless consideration is given to the manner in which we convey the expressed message. The *message treatment*, therefore, is the "decision . . . made in selecting and arranging both codes and content" [7]. Once these final decisions have been made, we must route the message across a *channel*. (See Figure 3.) Because the channel in the model involves the senses of hearing, seeing, touching, smelling, and tasting, the sensory channel selected must be appropriate to the message we wish to convey.

The receiver-decoder is one of the last links in our communication model. Behind the mask of a label is the person to whom the message is directed, that other individual who has been influenced by the same factors of communication, knowledge, attitudes, and sociocultural systems as we have been. Since no two people perceive an event or share their perceptions of that event in the same way, it is crucial to any verbal interaction that the receiver-decoder understands what we *mean* to convey. Our intent is not enough. We must aim for precision in our speech. The success with which we convey our thoughts determines how they will be absorbed and translated by the receiver-decoder. It is then up to him to provide us with some form of *feedback*, which allows us to determine the success or failure of our communication efforts.

Let us use an example to see how this model functions. While taking a walk in the vicinity of your neighborhood business area, an Oriental woman approaches you and asks you for directions (the referent). As the source-encoder, you need to rely on your knowledge of the area and your ability to communicate your knowledge. Your attitudes and awareness of sociocultural influences also affect your ability to give the requested information. Since the woman spoke to you in English, the *message code* you plan to use is English. You select your words with care, insuring clarity of expression (message content), and you speak slowly and distinctly (message treatment). The sensory channels you have chosen involve seeing and hearing. The woman must be able to *hear* your message and to see you as you speak and as you punctuate that speech with gestures.

Now you have given the directions *you* think the woman wanted, but does she think so?

As you are talking, the woman (receiver-decoder) listens intently and watches you as you point in the direction she is to go. She nods, repeats what you have

said, and states, "I think I'll be able to find it." The *feedback* she has given
you confirms that she perceived correctly the message you sent.

Another way of analyzing this verbal exchange is to compare it with Harold
Lasswell's verbal model. He asks:

> "Who?" (you, the source-encoder)
> "says what?" (the message, i.e., the directions)
> "in which channel?" (the sensory channels of hearing and seeing)
> "to whom?" (the Oriental woman, i.e., receiver-decoder)
> "with what effect?" (the Oriental woman thinks she can find her way;
> feedback) [8].

As we have seen in both examples, the use of models helps us analyze the
sequence of events when two people communicate. These events occur rapidly,
often simultaneously. Roles can interchange as well. For instance, the source-
encoder (i.e., the person who begins the verbal exchange) can also be the receiver-
decoder (i.e., the person who receives the message). Because of the rapidity of
exchange in a sequence of communication, and the interchanging of roles, we
can see how easily our model can distort the process when we consider only
one element to the exclusion of the others. Thus, to improve our communication it is necessary to examine each element *in relation to* the others in the
process.

If we select an inappropriate channel for our message, for instance, our purpose may not be accomplished because we may be unable to convey it correctly.
Berlo reiterates this by saying:

> The communication model . . . is all too easy to look at as a "click-click,
> push-pull" system. All communication ingredients . . . are intertwined.
> When we engage in communication as a process we cannot pull any one
> of them out or the whole structure collapses. When we want to analyze
> the communication process . . . we must remember what we are doing [9].

SUMMARY

Earlier we said that frustration is encountered with the prospect of having
to relearn communication skills used in nursing. Our discussion has been
focused upon the process involved when *any* two people communicate. A
visible form has been given to the process, which is called a model, and the
various elements in it have been identified as the referent, the source-encoder,
the message, the channel, the receiver-decoder, and feedback. All the elements
are operative and need to be examined in order to satisfy the curiosity we have
about our own communications.

The communication model, then, can be used to reexamine what we have
been doing, as well as to measure the ability we say we already have. Now we

must attach labels to a process we have used intuitively all our lives. By doing so, by really thinking about our basic communication, we will have begun a process essential to our profession. "Knowledge of the communication process itself affects communication behavior" [10]. This principle is basic, and its conscious application to our everyday interpersonal encounters should preface any further study of how we use our communication purposefully and beneficially in nursing.

NOTES

1. Miller, Gerald R. *Speech Communication: A Behavioral Approach*, p. 73.
2. Berlo, David K. *The Process of Communication*, p. 50.
3. Ibid., p. 54.
4. *The Oxford Universal Dictionary*, 3rd ed.; see the definition of *sentence*.
5. Berlo, op. cit. (note 2), p. 57.
6. Ibid., p. 59.
7. Ibid., p. 60.
8. Lasswell, Harold. *The Communication of Ideas*, p. 29.
9. Berlo, op. cit. (note 2), p. 69.
10. Ibid., pp. 48–49.

BIBLIOGRAPHY

Barnlund, Dean C. *Interpersonal Communication: Survey and Studies.* Boston: Houghton Mifflin, 1968.

Berlo, David K. *The Process of Communication.* New York: Holt, Rinehart and Winston, 1960.

Cherry, Colin. *On Human Communication.* New York: Wiley, 1957.

Goffman, Erving. *Behavior in Public Places.* New York: Macmillan, 1963.

Hyman, Ronald, ed. *Teaching: Vantage Points for Study.* Philadelphia: Lippincott, 1968.

Lasswell, Harold. The Structure and Function of Communication in Society. In L. Bryson, ed. *The Communication of Ideas.* New York: Harper, 1948.

Miller, Gerald R. *Speech Communication: A Behavioral Approach.* Indianapolis: Bobbs-Merrill, 1966.

Westley, Bruce, and MacLean, Malcolm. A Conceptual Model for Communications Research. *Journalism Quarterly,* 34:31, 1957.

Wiener, Norbert. *The Human Use of Human Beings: Cybernetics and Society.* Boston: Houghton Mifflin, 1954.

II

The Therapeutic Communication Model

2

The Nursing Event

THE BASIC COMMUNICATION MODEL discussed in Chapter 1 provides general information about what occurs when two people talk to each other through messages, channels, and feedback. This basic process is an incomplete foundation, because such communication has no aim except the mutual agreement or gratification of both parties, and although such end products serve as pleasant exchanges in friendships, they fall short of what is needed to accomplish a helping role with patients.

However, by taking the basic model in Figure 4 and supplying it with labels from nursing, we produce a model designed to help us relate the basic model to the therapeutic communication process. (See Figure 5.) Labels such as source-encoder and receiver-decoder now become recognizable identities — the nurse and the patient. The factors change only insofar as the purpose becomes more specific — in this case, meeting the needs of patients. Feedback tells us whether we registered, and also, in the therapeutic communication model, provides the information needed to evaluate the effectiveness of nursing actions.

What do we have? We have a visual means for studying the process involved in our attempts to direct our communication more specifically to individual patients. When any part of this process breaks down, the whole chain of events within it functions incorrectly. Our responsibility is to locate the specific difficulty within the process, and to examine and evaluate it in relation to the entire communicative interaction between ourselves and a patient.

Because of the visual nature of the therapeutic communication model we can examine abstract content along concrete pathways. It keeps us aware of the similar processes in our everyday communication and our purposeful

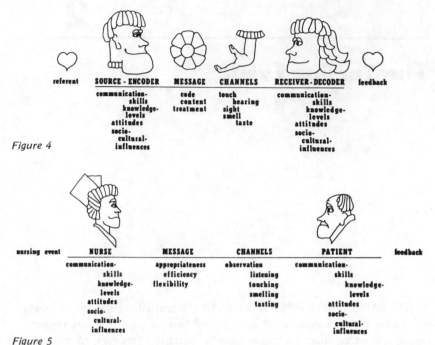

Figure 4

Figure 5

Figures 4 and 5. In Figure 4 (the same illustration appears as Figure 3 in Chapter 1) the basic communication model is shown. Figure 5, by the use of nursing labels, converts this design into a therapeutic communication model.

communication with patients. In addition, both models illustrate how we can build a therapeutic communicative approach from a process fundamental to all communication. Bearing in mind the similarities and differences between the two models, we can begin to examine and apply the components of the therapeutic communication model to our nursing experience.

THE REFERENT AS A NURSING EVENT

The term *referent* had been applied to a number of objects, acts, and situations occurring in human encounters. Now substitute the term *nursing event*, and to this more specific term attach all acts, situations, ideas, and experiences that directly activate our role as nurses with respect to the patients with whom we interact.

Who are our patients and where are they found? They are not limited to hospitals. During the course of our professional lives, the range of persons is as inclusive as it is diverse. It may be families with not enough to eat, or families whose members are obese. It may be a mother who delivered her ninth child, or a mother who has lost her first. It could be the dying old man who wants to live, or the husky teenager who wants to die. It could be the expressionless little girl living in a ghetto, old before her time, or the old woman wanting to be young again after her time. It could be all of these events many times over — people sick and needy on the one hand, and paradoxically healthy and resourceful on the other.

All these people require nursing care. In communities they are the "haves" and the "have nots" as far as health is concerned. Regardless of whether health needs are considered physical, mental, social, or spiritual, nursing efforts should encompass *all* of them. Nursing events cannot always be predicted, though they may be anticipated. Nevertheless, they will occur sometime in a hospital, in a family, or in a community, and given the opportunity, the skill, and the motivation, that is where nursing actions will be.

Components of the Therapeutic Communication Model

The Nurse as a Source-Encoder

IN ADDITION to our experiences in nursing we acquire a diversity of information, both concrete and abstract in content. In turn, this information must be applied to patient care situations with increasing ability and skill. Much can happen between the acquisition of knowledge and its application to patients, because in that interim we must learn to assimilate, plan, and distribute such information deliberately and effectively during interactions with patients.

Our source-encoding abilities increase dramatically as we begin to encounter patients and use the information we have acquired in our professional education. In the therapeutic communication model this information is divided into four major sections: our communication skills, knowledge levels, attitudes, and sociocultural influences.

The topics chosen for discussion in each of these sections have been elective choices, because the number of topics possible for discussion is unlimited in light of the continuing knowledge explosion, even in nursing. These topics represent areas of learning we need to consider further as we interact not only with our patients, but also with their families, in locales as traditional as the hospital, and as diverse and new as the community. It is for our patients, their families, and the many people we encounter within the community that we must explore the knowledge that extends beyond the basic information of nursing. Together these areas of learning become the source of our encoding abilities as professional nurses. The progressive security we achieve in becoming knowledgeable about these areas of learning also determines the extent to which we influence those with whom we interact. Influences that we communicate daily have, for our patients, far-reaching effects, which can facilitate or impede the kind and quality of nursing care we wish to give.

Introduction to Therapeutic Communication

WHAT IS THERAPEUTIC COMMUNICATION? Why use it at all? How is it supposed to enable us to help others better? Before these questions can be answered and the components of the therapeutic communication model can be discussed, let us look briefly at its development and some of the misunderstandings many of us have about this vital part of our nursing practice.

Approximately fifteen to twenty years ago therapeutic communication was not generally recognized as a vital clinical component of nursing curricula. Nurses were expected to confine their professional care of patients to more procedural or task-oriented activities. Talking to patients was something nurses did to fill in the silence while they were bathing patients — nothing more. Many nurses felt that taking additional time to talk to patients was not only an extravagant luxury, but also a waste of time. Good nurses were those who *did* something for or to their patients. This *something* was usually concrete and could be visibly appreciated by patients and nursing peers alike. Nurses engaging in deliberate conversation had a dubious reputation among their nursing colleagues, many of whom were convinced such actions would spoil patients and would result in overinvolvement with them.

Increased development and use of communication media brought us the realization that the influence of communication on our lives is pervasive and real. It is no less real for nursing. Steadily the inclusion of therapeutic communication into nursing programs became a reality. Each passing year increased our awareness that communicating with patients was not a nonchalant pastime, but the planned act of professionally responsible nurses. Even so, skepticism has continued. Nurses have seemed more eager to *do* than to seriously consider the *means* needed to *do*.

The abundance of articles on the subject has not lessened the outcry. Comments such as "All this psychological chitchat is for the birds," or "I came to be a nurse, and this (meaning therapeutic communication) isn't nursing!" are typical as the process of learning effective communication begins. These complaints are made before nursing knowledge and experience lend perspective to the varied roles and functions we have as nurses.

Putting frustrations about therapeutic communication aside, let us return to the purpose of such communication. Any nursing procedure, any act of reassurance, or any measure of comfort or relief, regardless of how small or seemingly incidental, is preceded by a form of communication. Every communicative act initiated in the presence of a patient has an impact on him. The effect of our communication style upon patients was not considered in the past, but it is now a part of our learning we cannot afford to waste. Each success or failure resulting from our nursing actions with patients indicates the effectiveness of the communication skills that have been consciously employed. The consistent efforts made in the use of these skills demonstrate to patients that their welfare is our primary concern.

The gap between communicating personally and professionally is wide. We thought the ability was innate until we started to learn about it from a therapeutic aspect. The resulting confusion and frustration necessitate a reclarification of what is meant by general and therapeutic communication.

Therapeutic communication requires planning so that one consciously influences less able persons into directions and actions beneficial to their welfare. The conscious act of planning suggests that personal communication styles are inappropriate because they are based on glibness, intuitive, unthinking responses, and mutual sharing between two people. These qualities cannot play a major role in an exchange that has as its primary objective the welfare of persons in need of assistance.

Definitions of therapeutic communication from various authors have in common these key words, *plan* and *consciously influence*, which should not be included in definitions of general communication. There are elements common to both types, but the key words should take precedence because through them our understanding of therapeutic communication increases and we come closer to actualizing its intent.

COMMON MISUNDERSTANDINGS

In the process of acquiring therapeutic communication skills, misunderstandings are likely. One misconception is that therapeutic communication is an artificial way of talking. Most of us are familiar with these and other comments that express such artificiality:

> "I'm so busy thinking about what I'm going to say, I don't feel I'm being myself."
> "I keep thinking my patient will be looking for the button that turns the sound track off."
> "It just doesn't sound like me."
> "I sound as though I'm using the words memorized from a script."

Many of us have had similar exchanges and encounters with patients, and we know how awkward they have been, and how poorly we have tolerated them. As a result, our ability to learn effective communication has been blocked temporarily.

There are no guarantees, no rules designed to eliminate these initial psychic discomforts. When therapeutic methods of communication are first implemented in dealing with patients, it is not uncommon to feel the process is artificial, especially when skill and precision are necessary. Identifying a particular skill and using it with precision require discipline, self-discipline that in all likelihood we have not been required to use before, let alone examine and evaluate. Being asked to implement this method of exchange in patient care settings or to share it in nursing conferences is often sufficient to increase anyone's frustration.

The need to excel, to succeed instantly, may be another factor contributing to the premise that therapeutic communication is artificial. Previous experiences in other schools, parental expectations, and our own self-concepts add to the stress of encounters with patients, and a sense of artificiality often is a byproduct. Therapeutic communication, in itself, is not synthetic; it is the medium of exchange between the helper and the helpless. The discipline required for this exchange to take place needs experiential time to mature before it becomes integrated into any communication that we wish to be effective.

Sometimes in the excitement of acquiring new knowledge (in this case, learning methods of therapeutic communication), we use these new methods in a variety of places with a variety of people, but most often with our nursing peers in clinical conferences and in class. These situations are appropriate for such use and function as the testing laboratory for becoming skillful in using other terms and phrases in the language of nursing. The resulting proficiency brings with it a greater sense of being a nurse — of professionally belonging. Great excitement and motivation accompany this feeling, especially when so much in nursing is new to us.

Each profession has its own vocabulary, one that fulfills the semantic needs of that profession alone. Learning that vocabulary is essential in order for us to function adequately within the profession.

The excitement with the newness of the vocabulary and the intensity of our nursing experiences very often increases the temptation to try communication techniques in various social settings. Take this example for instance:

A group of nursing students were invited to a party by the members of a law fraternity located on the campus. The party was enthusiastically received by the nursing students, who were still talking about it the next day. During a conference that day, one student gloated on the success she had had in using some of the therapeutic communication techniques on a law student. She felt she really came across well and was pleased by the law student's remarking on her conversational abilities. Other nursing students joined in with similar anecdotes in which their communication abilities had been noticed and felt they had been successful in conveying their new found skill to the law students.

This was not the appropriate time or place to practice therapeutic communication techniques, much less to use professional terminology. The vocabulary that increases our feelings of belonging professionally in one setting may well become the factor that sets us apart from people who are not nurses. Using techniques on other people, as the example illustrated, or talking about techniques in the presence of others, makes the conversation exclusive and private. The philosopher Ludwig Wittgenstein reaffirms this:

A language may be said to be private when it is devised to enable a limited number of persons to communicate with one another in a way that is not intelligible to anyone outside the group [1].

This exclusivity of conversation can foster another feeling. To others we become "those nurses" — that group of people who have little else to talk about except nursing.

Whenever we become involved conversationally with others in this manner, we are misusing therapeutic communication (not to mention other professional language). Such techniques, words, or phrases soon lose their meaning and value, and their professional impact is jeopardized. Words such as *meaningful relationship, dialogue, relatedness,* and even *therapeutic communication* have succumbed to ambiguous and humorous usage. Even within nursing they become professional fillers, which are substitutes for precise descriptive communication.

Other people, regardless of whether at parties, at lunch, or in dorms, are not our patients, and they do not necessarily know, like, or understand nursing. Every time we engage in professional banter (and often this is done automatically) at social events in the presence of people not in nursing, we shut them out, intimidate them with professional jargon, and cause them to seriously question whether we are capable of discussing other topics.

Our own dimensions as people will grow if we can remember that therapeutic communication is confined to nursing and our patients. When otherwise employed, the techniques can easily become an artificial and exclusive means to an end that is open to question.

A NURSING GOAL

All of us want to be proficient in the use of communication skills with our patients. Sometimes during our nursing practice, however, we become easily confused between directives to be therapeutic (or professional) and directives to be ourselves because we think of them as direct opposites. When this happens, being a therapeutic person means being different, and that difference is epitomized by the communication skills that are practiced in nursing.

Similarly, being ourselves may be interpreted as disregarding our responsibilities to our profession and to our patients. This confusion was very real to one nursing student who voiced her confusion in a conference shortly after caring for her patient, a 26-year-old woman with acute rheumatoid arthritis. She said, "I wasn't the least bit professional. As for being therapeutic, well, forget it." When this was discussed further, she related that she felt disgusted with herself because she had talked with her patient about skiing. The student discovered that she and her patient both enjoyed the sport, and she thought talking about it would distract the patient from the discomfort she was experiencing during the bathing procedure.

If the confusion between being therapeutic and being oneself continues, we are in danger of having to compromise in order to feel comfortable in the professional role. Then we become players; we assume a role that fits the situation. For example, if we interpret a nursing role as being impersonal or authoritarian, we may try to fit that interpretation. The psychologist Sidney Jourard discusses this professional charade:

> [There is a] difference between *taking* a role and *playing* a role. To take a role is a commitment to a task; to play a role is a charade. One reason a profession loses zest for its practitioners arises when the practitioner feels he can only work in a cut and dried, stereotyped way. [That] is why many nurses . . . ultimately get fed up with their profession. They lose zest because they feel that they have got to keep up the appearance of the role of a nurse . . . in some stereotyped way. When they do that what they are telling you is that they are more committed to imitating that role than they are in carrying out their professional commitment, that is [to] bring about results. When your commitment is to [your] goals and not means, you can't help but be eccentric, idiosyncratic, off-beat, oddball and creative [2].

Proficiency in communication does not mean preoccupation with techniques, which can easily happen, particularly in the initial phase of identifying and learning them. It is also not uncommon to feel intimidated by health professionals who favor a more orthodox communication approach to patients. Deviations or creativity may be discouraged or disregarded. When we become preoccupied with these factors, we lose our identities as individuals, not only to our co-workers, but also to our patients.

Feeling comfortable using these skills requires time, and it is then that the realization must come (if it is to come at all) that we are not parrots who mimic techniques to our patients, but intelligent and compassionate human beings who as nurses are trying to find and use a means of communication that will be effective with patients.

Mastery of technique should not become the ultimate objective in our efforts to communicate with patients or present us as being different from what we are. Being an oddball, an offbeat, or a creative person, as Jourard sees the committed professional, is something all nurses should risk. It is long overdue and it is needed, not only to perk up the profession, but also to bring more humanistic elements to patients.

The offbeat, creative person may reject the staid formalism of terms such as *therapeutic* in favor of a more novel approach, as did one nursing student who shared her definition of therapeutic communication with a group of peers: "What I'm being asked, in my opinion, is to do my own thing. Before I do it, however, I should be thinking about how it will affect my patient." This definition worked for her because both aspects of herself, as student and person, were involved in a way that took advantage of the best of each. As a student and as a person she could live with this approach honestly and still function effectively. According to Jourard, the blending produces an authentic person — someone who is "being oneself, honestly," in all human encounters [3].

Being real — being oneself honestly, for the benefit of patients — is the quality of the therapeutic nurse. We may use some techniques of therapeutic communication with success and we may discard others because they do not fit us or the situation with the patient. Regardless of these choices, we should be able to implement our intent to help by presenting ourselves to patients *as ourselves.* This is authenticity — this is real — and regardless of the label we use, this is the quality that translates an intent into the reality of a therapeutic nurse.

NOTES

1. Pitcher, George, ed. *Wittgenstein: The Philosophical Investigations,* p. 251.
2. Jourard, Sidney. *Disclosing Man to Himself,* pp. 70–71.
3. Jourard, Sidney. *The Transparent Self,* p. 133.

BIBLIOGRAPHY

Jourard, Sidney. *Disclosing Man to Himself.* Princeton, N.J.: Van Nostrand, 1969.
Jourard, Sidney. *The Transparent Self,* revised ed. Princeton, N.J.: Van Nostrand, Reinhold, 1971.
Pitcher, George, ed. *Wittgenstein: The Philosophical Investigations.* Garden City, N.Y.: Doubleday, 1966.

5

Communication Skills in the Nursing Interview

INTERVIEWING IS COMMON to every human interaction in which information is needed and shared. Though there are many types of information (such as facts and opinions) and many sources (such as television and radio), verbal interactions between people make interviewing a dynamic human experience. The giving and sharing of information between people has an eventual purpose, which, as Keltner observes, is determined by the people involved [1]. For example, to obtain information relative to a student's progress, a teacher may interview him. To learn how he performed on a written examination, a student may meet with a teacher. Other purposes requiring person-to-person encounters include problem-solving and decision-making (e.g., in medical, psychiatric, and counseling interviews), changing of beliefs or behaviors (e.g., in evaluation interviews, prisoner-of-war interrogations, and disciplinary interviews), and researching or discovering new information (e.g., in market interviews, questionnaire-controlled interviews, and police investigations) [2].

Interviews also take place in settings in which care of patients is involved, and most of them are between members of the health team; their function is to gather information, solve problems, make decisions, and do research *about* the patient that will facilitate and improve his care. These exchanges of professional information in turn contribute to the totality of health care for all patients.

The interview in nursing is the deliberate use of verbal behaviors by the nurse to communicate with the patient in a manner directly concerned with the restoration of his health. As such, these primarily verbal skills are central to the development of the professional nurse, because they assist in specifically identifying needs and help provide the basis from which to formulate and implement nursing goals relative to them. The intent of any helping relationship becomes clearer through the process of interviewing. Within this professional arena, the nurse counsels, assists, motivates, and shares pertinent information with the patient in a *mutual* effort to achieve the goals conducive to his recovery and well-being.

Every act of interviewing a patient should be a part of the total plan for nursing care, and each plan should contain general principles basic to the interviewing process. Principles are defined as fundamental truths that can be used to predict the consequences of a set of circumstances [3]. In nursing, the use of the interview based on such principles helps us to determine and reach our goals for nursing care. Whatever our nursing actions may be in an interview with a patient, they should incorporate these principles:

1. The freedom with which the patient expresses himself to the nurse is determined by the atmosphere the nurse creates in the presence of the patient.
2. An interview is effective to the degree that the nurse clearly establishes and understands the nursing goals in the interview.
3. An interview is effective to the degree that the nurse can relate to the patient without using value judgments.
4. An interview is effective to the degree that the nurse examines, encourages, and clarifies mutual thoughts and feelings that may affect nursing care.
5. An interview is effective to the degree the nurse consistently evaluates patient needs, nursing goals, and the behavioral responses of the patient to his nursing care.
6. An interview is effective to the degree that the nurse employs and encourages the use of feedback with patients in conveying, implementing, and evaluating nursing goals.

With these basic principles in mind, each time we employ interviewing skills with a patient, we reduce the unreliability and ambiguity of the information required to implement effective nursing care. Matters that are not related to the patient, his needs, and his care, that promote uncertainty, and that do not further the objectives of nursing care are extraneous to the aims of the interview.

The purposes of interviewing in nursing are specific to the patients' needs, but the types of information obtained from patients can be grouped into six general categories:

1. *Description*
   An account or a narration by the respondent of a happening in which he was a participant or a viewer.
2. *Perceptions*
   An account or explanation by the respondent of the extent and nature

of the information he has of the basic subject material, how much information he has and in what form he sees it.

3. *Behaviors*

   A determination of what the respondent did, what he does, what he will do, or what he has seen others doing.

4. *Attitudes and Beliefs*

   The identification of underlying assumptions or premises on which the respondent bases his comments and judgments.

5. *Feelings*

   The respondent's account of physical, emotional and other feelings as well as his revelation of these through his own physical reactions during the interview.

6. *Values*

   The respondent's revelation of those things that he considers good and bad, desirable or undesirable [4].

During an interview, to elicit any information that falls into these categories we need knowledge of the interviewing process, practice in its skills, and a conscientious and consistent evaluation of those skills. These elements provide a methodical and scientific framework on which to base our nursing activities, and they do not exclude the personal qualities of the nurse that make interviewing an art. There *is* room in the nurse—patient interview for spontaneity, warmth, and humor.

When nurses blend their own personalities and communication styles into interactions with patients, the interview becomes dynamic, changing, involved, and unique; in each instance the process is similar, but the experience is different. Every patient warrants the individual personality and communication style we bring with us, but these factors are of little value if they are not used in conjunction with the knowledge and methods of interviewing.

When we rely on our personality and communication style alone, we detract from and delay the plan of care patients need and have a right to expect from us. On the other hand, if we become preoccupied with interviewing methods or techniques, our approach to patients becomes mechanized. This also detracts from and delays effective nursing care, because it robs them of the individualized dimension nursing care should include.

Despite the abundance of literature on the subject, interviewing and interviewing methods cannot be learned from books alone. The value and effectiveness of these skills are entirely dependent upon how each of us uses them in interactions with patients. Time, practice, and patience — commodities not often found in those of us anxious to excel in being therapeutic with patients — are necessary to blend the knowledge of interviewing with our own personalities and communication style. We cannot use interviewing skills intelligently until we learn what those skills are, what guidelines exist for their use, and how to determine their effectiveness when they are used.

THE PURPOSE AND USE OF QUESTIONS

Questioning plays a major part in our daily communications. Its function is to produce some result during the course of a conversation — verify an expectation, clarify a point, or confirm an observation. The results obtained from our questions often hold more importance for us, however, than the process used in formulating them.

Those of us in nursing are no exception in wanting to see results from our interactions with patients, but no result of nursing efforts can be ascertained effectively unless we consistently examine the verbal means used to achieve such results. Questions invite, direct, and explore the verbal and nonverbal content offered us by the patient.

One purpose of interviewing mentioned earlier is to give and receive information. The nurse uses questions to acquire information needed to plan as well as to evaluate subsequent nursing care. The information received is as pertinent and specific as the question. Keltner states, "not only does an effective question stimulate the informant to share information, but it also provides him with some guide as to the nature of the information that is desired by the interviewer [5]. From the broad categories of information (i.e., description, perceptions, behaviors, attitudes and beliefs, feelings, and values) mentioned earlier, several general purposes of questions emerge. They are used to elicit responses with respect to the following points:

1. To describe and elaborate perceptions, ideas, and feelings
2. To clarify perceptions, ideas, and feelings
3. To validate observations
4. To substantiate facts
5. To assess the reliability of the information received
6. To interpret the meaning of a group of facts
7. To compare information with some predetermined criteria (e.g., nursing goals)
8. To formulate solutions based upon previous assessments and comparisons
9. To evaluate the outcome of a plan or action

These purposes can facilitate problem-solving in our nursing efforts because they increase the amount and accuracy of information we can use in determining subsequent nursing care. Asking questions for the purpose of collecting data is not enough if collection is the only reason for conducting the interview. The information must be relevant not only to the nursing goal, but also to the way that goal can be reached. In addition, it must be complete. Insufficient data result in faulty planning and insufficient nursing care. We cannot utilize information that we only think we have; we must be certain. Information gaps interrupt the therapeutic communication model's sequence of events. Questions provide us with one means to make certain that this sequence is complete.

OPEN-ENDED QUESTIONS

All of us use a variety of ways to set the tone and control the direction of our interviews with patients. Some of us arrange the chairs, adjust the lighting, and see that privacy is ensured. These are important steps, which are taken for the most part prior to the interview. The questions we employ also set the tone and control the direction of our interviews with patients. Open-ended questions are well-suited for initiating interviews because they do not restrict a patient's responses or confine him to a specific topic. He can respond in his own way to such questions, and it is from his individualistic response that we can begin to determine his attitudes and feelings, as well as to plan other questions that begin to touch upon his concerns.

The preliminary open-ended question gives each of us an opportunity to observe how the other person is responding verbally and nonverbally to the information being disclosed. These opportunities assist us in assessing the type and level of vocabulary used by the patient as he discusses a situation, event, or idea. Because open-ended questions elicit responses that are more than one or two words in length, they are well-suited to situations in which descriptive, elaborative, or comparative responses are needed. During these expanded responses the nurse can often determine the importance of the event to the patient, the chronological order of events, and the patient's frame of reference used in his observation of or participation in the event [6].

There are other advantages to using open-ended questions with patients in the interview. Through them, we convey more than just the question. We convey the feeling that we *care* about him, *care* about his thoughts and feelings, and *care* about the things he has to say, because *his well-being* is important to us.

The question and the interest and sincerity conveyed in it increase the patient's willingness to respond in a helpful, contributing manner, but do not force him to divulge information or recall an event before he is ready to do so. The feeling of having to supply an answer can be threatening to a patient and therefore inhibit his responses or force him to make up answers that will please us. The open-ended question allows him to verbalize in his own way. Given the opportunity, patients often voice their doubts and fears, as well as assist themselves in answering their own questions and in making their own decisions.

The patient's response to open-ended questions permits us to detect discrepancies or gaps in information. The knowledge supplied can be assessed and used to plan further questions that will give a more complete picture of his thoughts and feelings relative to his concerns and his nursing care.

Though open-ended questions allow patients freedom of response, they should be posed thoughtfully. Too many such questions or their exclusive use may cause the interview to be sidetracked by irrelevant topics. Overuse may also create confusion in both participants by clouding the original topic or point under discussion. With the abundance of information we can receive, we may have difficulty refocusing on the original topic or goals set for the interview. In addition, the information given in response to an open-ended question may, in some instances, be difficult to sort out.

Earlier, emphasis was placed on the importance of being ourselves and of using our own communication style, providing these two aspects are directed to the needs of our patients. From the practice and refinement of communication skills by health professionals in interview situations have come some common words that have proved useful not only in constructing open-ended questions, but also in facilitating the communication of our patients. The words *who, what, when, where,* and *how,* if used to introduce thoughtfully planned questions, guide communication, but they are not to be used without thought or relevancy. They are used only when the situation necessitates their use. They also can serve as a guide by which we can evaluate the effectiveness of our efforts to facilitate a patient's communication. They are valid when used thoughtfully and with due consideration for their purpose. Some examples of open-ended questions that illustrate this point are:

1. To describe and elaborate perceptions, ideas, and feelings.
   "What happened at your daughter's last night?"
   "What did she say that caused you to be upset?"
2. To compare the information with some predetermined criteria, such as nursing goals.
   "How does your former neighborhood in New York compare (or differ) from your present one here in San Francisco?"
   "In what way did your mother's behavior differ during her last visit?"
3. To formulate solutions based upon previous assessments and comparisons.
   "What plans have you made for your care when you leave the hospital?"
   "How might you deal with the situation if it should occur again?"
4. To assess the reliability of the information received.
   "What happened just before you received your pain medication?"
   "How many minutes went by between the time you asked for pain medication and when you received it?"
5. To evaluate the outcome of a plan or action.
   "What made your last visit to the senior center so enjoyable?"
   "What do you feel helped you do better on your last test?"

Like the opened door of a new house, open-ended questions introduce the nurse to the patient. His feelings, attitudes, ideas, and fears give him dimension much like the rooms we see in a new house. We cannot know what or who our patients are until we open the door with our questions and let them come in by means of their responses. The willingness of the patient to respond at all, much less completely, depends on how thoughtfully open-ended questions are used in an interview. Our obligation is to understand their purpose, to use them wisely, and to measure their effect by means of our patient's response to them.

CLOSED QUESTIONS

When we need specific information from a patient, we use closed questions. Just as open-ended questions encourage description and elaboration, closed questions elicit specific responses. For instance, the most common type of closed question such as "Are you tired?" or "May I sit next to you?" requires a yes or no response. They ask nothing beyond agreement or disagreement, and often the response can be given nonverbally with very little if any intrapersonal disclosure on the part of the patient.

Not all limited responses are as confined. Closed questions often require a patient to locate or identify a place or event pertinent to his situation. These questions are commonly used in health professions to gather data relating to the patient's discomfort and medical history. For example, in admitting a patient to a hospital (depending on his illness), using closed questions to learn his age, marital status, religion, allergies, and discomforts may be much more appropriate than saying, "Tell me something about yourself." These questions are a request for more disclosure than those requiring a yes or no response. They are exemplified by questions such as these:

"With which church are you affiliated?"
"When did you arrive at the doctor's office?"
"Where is your pain?"

Another way to limit a patient's response is to present him with two choices. For example:

"Would you like to get up now or in an hour?"
"Do you wish this injection to be given in your right or left arm?"

Though the choice is limited, the patient is allowed some part in making a decision. The implication is that we *expect* the patient to comply.

At the bedside, this approach is sometimes necessary, because patients do not always meet enthusiastically the tasks necessary for recovery. For instance, because of his physical discomfort, a patient may prefer not to move about on his first postoperative day for fear that his pain will be aggravated. He may understandably decline if we ask "Would you like to get out of bed?" Having given him the choice, we must either honor the patient's wishes made in the response or alter our question so that his choice is limited to the expectations of his treatment plan.

Questions allowing limited choice are particularly important when working with children. Not only do we lessen the risk of the child saying no, but we also provide him with a means to become autonomous. For people who are indecisive, depressed, or highly anxious, the security offered in the structure of a limited choice question gives them a feeling of accomplishment through their participation in decision-making, regardless of how small it may be.

Often patients with a limited vocabulary, minimal education, or lack of culturally enriching experiences are more comfortable in responding to closed questions [7]. Not only do they know what is expected in the question, but they also feel they are contributing to their care. Conversely their discomfort with the overuse of broader questions results from not knowing precisely what is expected of them. From this uncertainty springs a fear of betraying their lack of knowledge when responding. Consideration for the patients' verbal *ability* to share information with us must be foremost in guiding us in the planning of our questions — especially closed questions.

Despite the limited scope of closed questions, the responses are often not as limited as they appear. People usually qualify their answers, *as if* responding to an open-ended question, thereby giving more information than requested. Some examples from various nurse-patient interactions illustrate this point:

> *Nurse:* Did your neighbor in the next apartment move?
> *Patient:* No, he's in big trouble though. He hasn't paid his rent for five months now. The police are coming today to evict him. He's big trouble.

> *N:.rse:* Do you like the stories you've read?
> *Patient:* No! I guess it's just because of my curiosity. I get started reading them and then I can't put them down. Besides, these stories always leave off at an exciting place and you die until you find out what happens in the next issue.

> *Nurse:* Did you have a nice weekend?
> *Patient:* Oh yes. I went to visit my brother in Anaheim on Saturday. We went to Marineland Sunday and had a great time.

As we can see, the responses contain more information than asked for in the questions.

Let us examine additional responses to closed questions drawn from other nurse-patient interviews. In looking at these responses, try to construct questions that would have elicited the elaborations.

> *Response:* I don't drink much milk. My stomach can't take it. My doctor took me off it a long time ago.
> *Response:* No, my relatives are all dead except for some second cousins back East.
> *Response:* I'm not sure, but I think you come to visit us old-timers to see how we live in this community.

Rephrasing questions to exclude these elaborative or descriptive responses points to the need to give more thought to their use. If we get the same elabor-

ative responses with closed and open-ended questions, we can see how difficult
it is to correctly phrase them.

Previously, we discussed the way closed questions are used with validity in
nurse-patient interactions, but their limited advantages must not overshadow
some of their disadvantages. When closed questions are used in an interview,
they tend to block the free flow and exchange of communication, especially
if they are used as the primary means for collecting information from the patient.

In initial interviews, and in situations in which we feel personally under stress,
we tend to rely more heavily on closed questions. At these times, such an
approach represents safety; we can obtain the necessary data and retreat. For
those of us who do not always feel at ease communicating with patients or are
shy with them, such questions help initiate verbal activity, even though it is
limited. To others of us, they can be used to obtain information quickly,
without much thought. Such expediency does not promote empathetic relationships.

Closed questions are easy to ask. We do it all the time. They are therefore,
a source of instant gratification in our interactions with patients. They make
us sound more knowledgeable without exposing a lack of flexibility and communicative planning in talking with patients. Overuse of these specific and
restricted questions threatens the ease with which a patient may wish to respond.

When we depend on these questions we run the risk of conveying to our
patient that we are too busy to listen to him, that the information we receive
is more important than the person giving it, or that we do not wish to facilitate
a helpful exchange of communication. He may think that anything he says is
inconsequential. Faced with these possibilities, we can understand why patients
may feel dehumanized in interactions with us and other health professionals.

Closed questions cannot and should not be eliminated from an interview;
avoiding their use is impractical and unrealistic. Though they are limited in
scope, when used *carefully,* they supplement the other types of questions and
communication approaches possible in interviewing patients.

LEADING QUESTIONS

Leading questions are closed questions that restrict the patient's response
because they contain a suggestion. An expectation is implied, as in most questions, but in this case it is often posed to meet the needs or goals of the nurse.
The implication is not *an* expectation, but *the* expectation of what the answer
should be relative to the patient and his situation. The following example
illustrates this point:

> A student had been visiting an elderly lady as part of her community
> nursing experience. During the course of the conversation, Mrs. M. re-
> called to the student that she had decided to go to the afternoon showing

at a neighborhood theater without checking to see what movie was scheduled. Once inside and seated, she discovered that the film was an adult movie, and after viewing it for several minutes, she decided to leave. After she recounted this, the student responded by asking, "Didn't you find that type of movie disgusting?" Mrs. M. replied, "Not at all. Even though the movie didn't interest me, I wasn't disgusted by it."

The woman's response to the question was the opposite of what was *expected*. The student was expressing her own personal value judgment rather than first seeking to elicit a description from the woman. In this instance, she placed the woman in the position of having to defend her actions and thoughts.

Because the answer is implied in a leading question, the patient is led to a particular response — one of our own choosing. Certainly an expectation is a legitimate goal in posing a question, but only if the patient is given the right to choose the expectation he wishes to meet. Any question should allow a reply without intimidation or defensiveness. Although we may not like the answer, we have at least allowed the patient the freedom of choice.

In addition to the value judgments in leading questions, two other factors may distort a patient's response and they become evident in queries that challenge a patient or contain emotionally charged words. Both types can produce a reaction rather than a thoughtful, accurate reply.

Challenging a patient in terms of motivating him to function constructively is helpful, but posing questions that cast doubt on his integrity or capabilities as an individual is not beneficial. Likewise, stimulating discussion on the basis of thought and reason can be rewarding in an interview, but doing so on the basis of emotional appeal is not. We are not engaged in nursing practice to challenge our patients' integrity or ego-identity, and we should not be using an interviewing situation to prove how wrong the patient is and how right we are. Few of us impose our standards upon patients deliberately, and this makes the use of leading questions difficult to understand. We use them when we communicate with our friends in other settings, and there they are accepted as a matter of course.

Leading questions that contain emotionally charged words may precipitate the opposite reaction from what we expect. We saw in the previous example that the word *disgusting* has emotionally charged overtones. Questioning with these words often appears to be an attack on a patient's values and beliefs. Consequently, these are not as likely to be discussed calmly. Emotion-evoking terms are used frequently on television — in jest, satire, or derision — to get a reaction from the audience. Think how they may likewise cause a patient to react even though implemented unwittingly. In the process we may undo many of our helping efforts made on their behalf.

The following examples illustrate some of the controversial, often upsetting, questions that are charged with challenge, emotion, and opinion:

"You *aren't* going to stay in bed again, are you?"

"Do you think your doctor was *wise* in allowing you to get out of bed so soon?"

"You are going to change that *smelly* undershirt before our interview, aren't you?"

"Don't you think Catholics are *smart* enough to function independent of Rome?"

"You mean you think *all* men with long hair are no good?"

"*How* do you know you're so right?"

"I imagine you'll be pretty sad when my visits with you come to an end, won't you?"

Patients are our most immediate source of feedback when we use leading questions, because their responses can be revealing. The raised eyebrow, the surprised, hurt look, or the tightened appearance around the mouth may often indicate a reaction of anger. In the midst of such expressive behaviors, we soon begin to see the negative influence our leading questions, with their overtones of challenge, emotion, and opinion, have upon our patients.

Despite the negative effects leading questions may have, they may not always be interpreted as such by all our patients. Strongly implied biases may be deflected because of our rapport with them, our sincerity and concern overriding obvious, negative implications. Such qualities, however, are not substitutes for thoughtfully directing our questions along less disputable lines. Controversies will always be with us, as will impulsive opinions in our comments and questions. Both are hard to avoid, even with the best of intentions, but we must try, and we can begin by limiting the use of leading questions.

THE USE OF SILENCE

Why is silence so uncomfortable? Why will we do almost anything to avoid a period of silence in our interviews with patients? The two-second lull seems more like two excruciatingly long hours, and the prospect of this long wait often impels us to fill the void with words. Learning to be comfortable with silence is one of the most difficult skills to accomplish in our interactions with patients.

Conversation is a highly prized ritual in our society. All of us are judged by how often and to what extent we express ourselves. Talking is as much a *doing* task in nursing as are emptying bedpans, giving baths, and administering injections. Talking is activity, functioning, something that can be measured because it elicits a response from the patient. Talking is getting answers, results, cooperation. In our contemporary society, social acceptability depends in large part on our ability to relate to others. We do not have time for the person who cannot express himself well or in the same manner as ourselves. Those who can articulate are "in," and those who cannot are "out." Nursing does not differ in this respect; it too demands effective expression. Verbal ability is emphasized and silence de-emphasized as a skill in nursing, but both are important.

In the framework of the interview, silence can be defined as the period of time during which the nurse waits without interruption for the patient to begin or resume speaking [8]. Do not assume, however, that this means that silence is passivity, or that it represents a lack of interviewing skills. On the contrary, activity is taking place, but it is not overt. Silence marks the conclusion of our vocalizations, and it gives us an opportunity to sift and sort the thoughts we have absorbed and file them for later use.

Silence has always been a part of our lives, and as such has been alternately comforting and disturbing. Our moments of quiet have provoked thought, helped us find solutions to problems, afforded us calmness and privacy, and conveyed our displeasure, our hurts, and our approval to others. It encompasses a variety of moods common to ourselves and to our patients. The similarities of these moods can assist us in understanding what a patient is trying to convey through his silence, as well as in acquiring skill in the use of silence when we are with him.

There are two things to consider about silence: its function in the interview process and the problems encountered through its use. We said previously that it allows us to think, to sift our ideas, and to plan how they will be used. These functions are important in our interviews with patients, because silence usually is the natural conclusion of a logical sequence of thoughts within the discussion. These interludes can be used for the reflection of our thoughts and the formulation of an alternate approach when the interview continues.

Periods of silence give us an opportunity to observe our patients unobtrusively. Does he seem comfortable? What type of silence is being conveyed during these periods? Is it one of thoughtfulness or anger and resistance? Does the patient seem to be having difficulty in answering? How is he responding nonverbally to our comments and questions? Often these cues are significant and should be considered when we wish to validate our observations during silence.

Another function of silence is to invite a response. Doing so with comfort not only encourages verbal communication, but also conveys an expectation to our patients that they *can* respond if given the needed time to formulate an answer. This time period differs among patients; not all of them can reply quickly or have a large vocabulary from which to draw. Older people, for example, regardless of their health status, need added time because their physical and mental processes become slower with age. We must, therefore, promote an accepting silence that conveys our faith in their ability and strength to respond. Impatience on our part can frustrate their efforts, and the final verbalization can become garbled and misunderstood. As a result, each ensuing episode becomes more upsetting until the incentive to communicate is gone. Furthermore, during silence, a patient can recollect thoughts and events, appraise them, and decide on a course of verbal action. A rapid pace in the interview does not allow for these thought processes to become actualized.

Another function of silence is to allow us to assess the level of anxiety in ourselves and our patients. Such a determination is important because the ability to communicate intelligently and effectively is influenced by the degree of anxiety experienced by the participants. Depending on the topic under discussion in the interview, anxiety levels can change several times. If the levels in either ourselves or our patients become too high, communication can be severely reduced or blocked. If we observe and assess the early signs of anxiety during silence, intervention is possible *before* it impedes the course of the interview. Such attempts not only ease interpersonal strains, but also direct the psychic energies into more verbally constructive channels. Such an assessment was made by the nursing student in the following example:

The day before this conversation I noticed an aversion in myself to talking with M. I couldn't sit with her for more than five minutes and I squirmed the whole time. That night I analyzed my behavior and came to the conclusion that in my anxiety, I had become too impatient with M. My original goals were too high, and because they were, I became frustrated. I had been having trouble allowing her to verbalize and realized that I had begun to push too hard. I went into this interview feeling more calm and with the intention of using therapeutic silence to convey my willingness to have her take her time in expressing herself verbally.

Nurse: Hello, M. Shall we sit over here where it's quiet? [I did this so that there would be no diversions of our attention.]
Patient: Okay.

We sat down. There followed a silence of about two minutes. My hands were folded in my lap. I was acutely aware of the silence; every sound seemed intense. Then M. shifted her weight in the chair, and the sound seemed very loud. I was just hoping that she would say something. My heart was beating faster than usual.

Patient: Is it raining out today? [She was sitting stiffly in her chair. She glanced at me.]
Nurse: No. It's cold, but it looks like it will rain later. [I was relieved that she said something. I was almost exhilarated and felt like laughing.]

There was silence for another three minutes. During this time she kept looking at me. I felt she was checking to see if I was tense. This time, however, I didn't feel particularly tense, and I smiled at her during the silent intervals. Soon after this interval she brought up a topic and continued to discuss it until we were interrupted by another patient. I felt my ability to relax during these silences was beneficial to M. I can see now how my anxiety must have affected her and how a person can "push too hard" even trying to endure a silence. Whatever direction M. takes during our times together is very much influenced by me. I never realized that until now and can see the difference that my anxiety made in my previous interviews with her.

The comfort experienced by the nursing student during the silence in this interaction resulted from her recognition of nonverbal cues as an indication of the patient's readiness to converse and her ability to assess and control her own anxiety in order to facilitate verbal communication.

Silence at crucial intervals during our interactions with patients does not mean the absence of activity. To maintain a comforting yet facilitating silence we must use actions and sounds to demonstrate our acceptance of patients. The way we sit and the way we use our bodies communicate this attitude. Sounds of encouragement, such as "uh-huh," and "hm," are often helpful. They are vocal byproducts of silence; they neither demand nor interrupt.

Despite its beneficial aspects, we cannot all be comfortable in a silent situation. Most of us *want* to be comfortable, but our own needs, values, and discomforts get in the way. These are common problems all of us have experienced at some moment of silence with our patients.

A frequent source of difficulty in maintaining an accepting silence is our inability to incorporate it into the tempo of the interview. We are often made aware of the pace by the way a patient verbally responds to our questions. If our inquiries are geared to obtaining the information we need, the interview moves along until its conclusion.

The quickness or successfulness with which the interview is terminated depends upon the patient's ability and willingness to verbally respond. Age, culture, understanding, and levels of knowledge affect the pace of the patient's communication. Adapting to his *verbal* tempo is not as disconcerting or as difficult for us as is adapting to the way he may pace his periods of silence.

When we assess the expressive communication patterns of any patient, the patterns and use of silence should be included. Once this is established, we can not only plan how to use them in our interview, but we can also adjust more comfortably to the idea that silence is useful and plays an important role in our interactions with patients. This accomplishment alone can help us gain insight into the nature of the helping relationship. Such a discovery was made by the nursing student in the following example:

> I used to think that in most relationships started by two strangers, initial silences would be long and frequent, then diminish as they got to know each other. In my relationship with Mrs. B., however, the opposite is true. In our very first visits there was never a moment of silence, either by natural inclination or in the therapeutic sense. But now, and particularly in my most recent visit, the silent periods seem to be cropping up more and more. Sometimes they are reflective, such as after we talked about her husband's death, but mostly they are relaxed silences in which we contemplate things we had said.
>
> This new development in seeing how silences can work and how comfortable I can be in them actually makes me excited and proud of what I

have been able to accomplish. The entire aspect and atmosphere of my visits is changing and the pleasant and sometimes superficial chats we had developed into a feeling of closeness and the discussion of some really *heavy* ideas! Both of us need a moment or two of silence to digest what has just been said. What a great way to get rid of the cobwebs in my thinking!

Extremes of silence also create problems. We can use too much or not enough when we are with our patients. What is too much silence? It is the prolongment of the period of time during which one waits for a response or a continuation of a topic to a point of noticeable discomfort. Prolonged silence occurs when we have misperceived our patient's readiness to respond. When this happens, both participants have misunderstood the expectations of the interview or the communication preceding the silence.

Although an occasional period of prolonged silence may not inhibit the interview, our anxiety level begins to rise as the periods become more frequent or more prolonged. Because our expectations have not been understood, our anxiety begins to be communicated by behaviors that further inhibit the course of the interview. These behaviors may take the form of "sitting it out," or of our patients' use of repetition in order to reorient us to their previous remarks or anger, frustration, and defensiveness. There may be many more ways of indicating frustration during this time, but the point is that the overuse of silence and the behaviors that are likely to result from it do not advance communication along helping channels.

Perhaps the person having the most difficulty with the overuse of silence is the nurse who by nature is quiet, shy, or taciturn. Combined with these personality tendencies, silence becomes a communicative extension of the nurse in interpersonal relationships with patients. Though there are many instances in which a natural comfort with silence is a therapeutic asset in that it is readily conveyed to the patient, it can also be a liability when verbal participation is expected in the interview. This factor alone often leads to unfortunate misunderstandings and misinterpretations by patients and co-workers.

It is essential that those of us who are more comfortable with silence than verbosity carefully assess not only our patterns of communication, but also the effect *our silence* might have upon our patients. In the process of self-evaluation, our patients often serve as our most immediate sources of feedback. If they consistently convey discomfort during silent periods, an immediate reassessment is needed, and it should involve returning to the therapeutic communication model to locate the miscommunication so that an alteration can be made in the sequence of our communication.

Infrequent silence, on the other hand, can also have an adverse effect during an interview, primarily because of our inability to perceive how silence is being used by the patient. When we misinterpret its use, we take action to minimize or shorten it during interviews. One common action is interruption. In a conversation, this occurs ordinarily when one person interjects comments before the other person finishes speaking. Gorden reminds us that interruptions are not necessarily limited to verbal expressions; they can be any behavior that prematurely distracts a patient's thinking or interrupts his readiness to continue with the interview [9]. The finality with which he ends his comments, nonverbal behaviors (such as an expectant gaze), even verbal comments that he is ready to proceed are cues to watch for during interviews.

Our own discomfort with silence reduces our ability to perceive what is communicated by a patient's silence. Our ability to be verbally expressive may limit our ability to use silence effectively. As discussed previously, today's world is an articulate world. Our expectations of others are based upon these standards for articulation. Many patients willingly meet these requirements, reinforcing our expectations of future patients.

Use of these standards in helping relationships can diminish our effectiveness. If we expect our patient to express himself as easily as we do, the outcome for us can only be frustration. When a patient does not fit our verbal mold, he runs the risk of being labeled as aloof, distant, and uncooperative.

Because a patient may have different communication patterns and through that difference be considered unproductive, our own anxieties begin to enter into our interactions with him. We miss his cues and the mood of his silence by our interruptive verbal and nonverbal insistence that his response be equal to our questions or meet our expectations. If a silence continues too long on the basis of our anxious perceptions, we assume that our patient has not understood us and immediately rephrase the question or change the topic. This occurs so rapidly and subtly that many of us do not realize that perhaps only two or three seconds have elapsed — hardly enough time for anyone, much less a patient, to absorb the meaning, formulate a reply, and respond to a question or comment. This is further corroborated in various studies, which have revealed that as silence increases it is more than likely to be interrupted by the person conducting the interview [10]. The implication is that the effective use of silence rests primarily with us.

Being comfortable and helpful during silence with our patients and using it to promote thought, acceptance, and further verbal participation, *is learned* only by practice during our encounters with patients. More often than not, it is achieved by making mistakes in assessment, in pacing and timing, and in the perception of our own comfort and of how a patient is using silence. We often learn more by making mistakes than by doing things perfectly.

In these situations, learning involves consistent evaluation of the effect silence has upon the patient. Often we are so busy trying to achieve a goal or a grade through use of a specific technique that we fail to observe the variety of moods a patient can communicate during these periods. These efforts contradict our desire to be ourselves. What must be learned is patience, and with it, the desire to know our patients and their communication through the medium of silence.

TACTICS OF CLARIFICATION

No interview can progress very far unless both participants are sure they understand what has been said. Any groundwork that has been prepared in previous interviews will disintegrate if we proceed too far without seeking clarification. Information obtained without it is likely to become an assumption, which can only lead to misunderstandings and ineffective nursing care.

With the increasing need for accurate information in health settings, the need for us to understand clearly the information we have and to seek clarification whenever we do not understand becomes paramount. The task of achieving it can seem endlessly repetitive and thankless. If we look at the skill more closely, however, we see that what may seem repetitive need not be, and that it may seem thankless due to our limited ability to see the ways in which it can be used.

The ability to clarify is a versatile skill because it can be used so many ways with our patients. Human communication can be imprecise, rambling, and unrelated in varying degrees at different times. Inclusive terms (such as *they* and *them*), ambiguous phrases (such as *you know*), and words with double meanings (such as *stoned* and *trip*) can easily create confusion.

Use of one communication approach for all clarification needs is too static in helping relationships that are always changing. One aspect of helping relationships does not change, however. We *must* understand what is being said by our patients, and we must assist them to understand anything that may not seem clear to them. *How* we achieve that is dependent upon the techniques available to us and the different ways they can be used.

When we request clarification, we are asking for clear, specific information that elaborates upon a vague, ambiguous, or implied statement made previously by the patient in our interview [11]. Whenever we attempt clarification to ensure understanding or agreement between ourselves and our patients, we are using it as a specific therapeutic communication approach.

Richardson suggests that since clarification is used when we are not expecting the response we get, improvement in planning our questions is indicated. When we investigate the ways we can develop our ability to clarify and employ this variety actively and deliberately in our interviews, we are using a tactic — an approach that is planned. In this book, *tactic* is offered as a word implying variety not only in seeking different methods in the development of our ability to clarify, but also in all communication approaches with our patients. If we seek clarification by using examples, by pointing out omissions and inconsistencies, by identifying similarities and differences, by questioning meaning, and by restating, reflecting, and summarizing, we can improve our interviews.

Clarifying by Example

Sometimes we are unable to understand a point being conveyed by another person, and examples bring clarity into the discussion by linking the abstract or vague conversational point to a specific or concrete illustration. Many of us do this already, and it has become integrated into our own conversational style. Examples are used in the classroom and on educational television, where their impact is often greater visually than verbally.

In nursing, there are many situations in which examples have an important clarifying function. Instructing the diabetic patient about injections, the ulcer patient about his diet, and the colostomy patient about self-care are just a few. Implicit in the use of examples is that they convey the clarity intended. This presupposes that they are relevant to the point needing clarification.

This means of clarifying usually indicates how well we understand others. Patients sometimes are less intimidated by our jargon and knowledge if we translate what we know into a practical and understandable example, using words that are familiar to them.

If we are not sure of a point a patient may be trying to make, we can ask him for an example. With the example and the original point of discussion, we may have enough information to reiterate what he has been trying to say. In the process we may lessen his concern about having to repeat himself in order to be understood.

Identifying Omissions and Inconsistencies

In his eagerness to convey his ideas or relate an event to us, a patient may leave out things, or his statements may seem inconsistent with what he said previously. We must not assume that our perceptions of these apparent omissions and inconsistencies are true — they must be substantiated. In pointing them out during an interview, we should encourage the patient to supply the information needed to complete his communication.

In busy hospital and clinic settings it is very hard for any patient to remember details. Likewise, older people and children sometimes forget a sequence of events during their discussions with us. The task for us here is to express to the patient that something might be missing from the events he is relating to us. Sometimes reverbalizing the sequence helps him realize the omissions or inconsistencies and allows him to continue. At other times, just expressing our confusion with the sequence as it has been related to us refreshes his memory and makes the events he has discussed seem more orderly and understandable.

Identifying Similarities and Differences

Each interview builds on the one preceding it. In the course of examining the information we have received, certain patterns begin to form. From them we know how a patient thinks and how he interacts with those about him. The similarities and differences in these patterns can be determined through an assessment of various interviews, and from them, future interviews can be planned.

Once established, these patterns can help us clarify events in future interviews. Assisting a patient to identify the similarities or differences of his discussion or experience can facilitate his problem-solving abilities. Identification of similarities necessitates recall of positive or negative experiences. Helping a patient see the similarities of positive events can reinforce his self-esteem and his self-confidence. Likewise, with events having a negative effect, a patient can see the recurrent theme that may be creating a problem for him.

The identification of differences in a patient's experiences can assist him in learning ways to constructively deal with uncomfortable or difficult interpersonal situations so that he can avoid a repetition in future experiences. Approaches such as "In what ways was this experience similar?" or "How was this experience different?" may promote a better understanding of a situation or a conversation for both ourselves and our patients.

Clarifying by Questions

Incidents that do not lend themselves to examples or comparisons are best dealt with directly by asking the patient what he means about the things he is saying. Questions such as "What do you mean?" and statements such as "I don't understand what you mean" notify a patient that we may not be perceiving his remarks correctly and that elaboration is necessary before the interview can proceed. This does not mean that our approaches should be used in a challenging manner. By strongly emphasizing specific words in our questions, we can alter what we are trying to convey. Again, this tactic of clarification can act as a stimulus to the patient and facilitate a more precise or elaborative response.

Clarifying by Restatement and Reflection

Restatement and reflection, as clarifying techniques, are used to relay our understanding of a patient's comments. Though both techniques facilitate clarification, each does so differently, and both can become easily confused if these differences are not fully understood.

Restatement requires that we reformulate *in our own words* what we think the patient has said. This sets into motion a validation process that, when achieved, allows the interview to proceed. Interspersed throughout the interview are our efforts not only to check the validity of our understanding with the patient, but also to achieve an on-the-spot clarification from him. The aim of this approach is validation through clarification; the means used is restatement.

No new information is being sought at these times. Validity, clarity, and understanding of the old (i.e., previous) information are the major aims of the use of this skill.

Often when we engage in restatement, we preface our remarks with the phrase "In other words." Here we are verbally indicating to the patient that we plan to translate what he has said into our own words. If we do this successfully, we confirm to ourselves and to him that we have understood *because we have translated that knowledge into other words,* which in turn have been understood by him. Other prefacing statements such as "If I understand you correctly . . ." or "Let me see if I have this right . . ." may also be used. The variety of ways by which each of us conveys this translation is endless, and we should use variety because people in need are different, as are their ways of speaking. By trying to develop variety in restatement, as in all communication skills, each of us can more ably demonstrate his interest and intent to begin at the patient's own ability level.

Reflection, on the other hand, creates much more confusion, not only in application, but also in recognition of it as a clarifying tactic separate from restatement. Reflection means repeating the patient's words *as he says them* (sometimes called echoing), either in part or in whole. The words are reflected to him much as a mirror reflects the exact image of the person who is looking into it. The purpose is to assist him in the exploration of his own reasoning, and it is facilitated through echoing the sentence or phrase *he has just said.* In this respect, as Richardson proposes, reflection allows us to gain *additional* information that may help us in assisting the patient [12]. This type of reflection is called the reflection of *content* because we are dealing and responding to the *words* of the patient.

A common error made in the use of reflecting content involves the definition of the word *reflect.* There is a great temptation to use *reflect* as it is defined through popular usage — to look back thoughtfully over what has taken place. Instead, we are using it to mean the echoing of the patient's words. If we reflect by simply thinking over events and conversation, we have taken too much leeway in interpreting what the patient has said. The reflection of content requires only that the words be used in echoing to the patient what he has said so that he can become more involved in the elaboration.

Another common error in the use of reflecting content is its indiscriminate overuse. It became popular when introduced by psychologist Carl Rogers, and repetitive echoing seemed to dominate interview situations. Reflecting content became a blocking agent because patients misinterpreted it as mimicry. None of us would do this consciously to any patient, but echoing bounces back upon him. This skill in particular needs to be used in conjunction with other skills in order to achieve maximal effect with patients. Then it is a useful tactical communication approach. Used exclusively, it can generate antagonism and frustration from our patients.

Echoing of words or phrases is not the only type of reflection used for clarification. Many times patients' feelings and thoughts are conveyed nonverbally and through impressions that do not always correspond to the words being spoken. They may not always realize how expressive they are or their need to share what they are feeling and thinking. When we perceive something is bothering a patient, we often remark to ourselves, "He sounds upset," or "She looks sad," or "He's got something on his mind." By affording him an opportunity to share these unspoken yet communicated thoughts and feelings, we employ another type of reflection, namely, the *reflection of feeling*.

This type of reflection is a communication skill that gives us an opportunity to clarify unspoken or incongruent impressions we are receiving from patients. There are many ways of approaching the feeling content in a patient's communication. One way is by incorporating what we have taken in with our senses and verbalizing our impressions with phrases such as "You sound pleased" and "You look sad." Another approach may be to point out gently the apparent contradiction between what a patient is saying and what he is conveying nonverbally. For example, "You say you're happy with the outcome of your biopsy, but you don't look happy with the report." Such comparisons afford us the opportunity to achieve clarification by requesting that the patient verify whether or not what we saw and heard was accurate. This, in turn, may be enough to stimulate him to explore feelings that he may need to examine and share.

The difficulty in using this skill is that we are dealing with another person's feelings, and what may seem predictable one day is unpredictable the next. A person who may seem to be master of his feelings may fall apart over a seemingly trivial matter. We can never really be sure of what feelings we are dealing with even when we are with our patients over a period of time.

Prolonged stress, family relationships, job worries, and early childhood influences all play a part in how our patients act and feel when we encounter them. We cannot, nor should we, plunge into a patient's reservoir of feelings simply to take the plunge. It is not an appropriate justification for any nursing action, because we may be unable to deal with the feelings we pursue. These are actions that none of us wish to inflict upon our patients.

When we attempt to clarify the feelings a patient may be conveying, we should consider our rapport with that patient and the manner in which he uses his words. Rapport is the first consideration because it implies a basic trust, comfort, and security between us. It provides the interpersonal base from which to pursue other nursing actions. Rapport is not developed overnight, but on the other hand, it does not take months.

An assessment of the way patients use their words is also important. Many times we find that a word, such as *angry*, may be unacceptable for some patients, because to *them* it evokes feelings of violence, loss of control, or helplessness. To be angry therefore is not a part of *their* behavior as *they* see it. These people may have acceptable substitutes for that feeling — words such as *annoyed, irritated,* or *out of sorts.* If this is the case, it would be preferable for us to use them in any attempt to clarify patient's feelings through reflection.

Developing skill in using the reflection of feeling requires sensitivity to our patients' feelings. A guideline that may help in developing this skill is to confine its use to the immediacy of the "here and now," that is, dealing with patients as they present themselves to us in situations in which we encounter them. These situations provide us with enough opportunities to assist them without delving or probing into their past personal experiences, especially those that are not germane to the situation at hand.

Even in present situations, not all patients can or are ready to express their feelings. They should not be forced to do so if their emotional equilibrium may be disrupted in the process, or if their overall nursing care may be adversely affected. Nevertheless, many patients welcome the opportunity to share their feelings with us. They are quick to notice the constant activity we are engaged in when in clinic and hospital settings and the high case loads of nurses working in the community. Often the only way they know we care and are interested is when we verbalize our impressions of what they appear to be experiencing and feeling.

Let us look at the differences between restatement and reflection again. In restatement we use *our own words* to validate what a patient has just said — to clarify the meaning and accuracy of *old* information. In reflection, on the other hand, we explore *new* information in two ways: by the reflection of content in which we echo to the patient *his own words,* either in part or in whole, or by the reflection of feelings in which we put into words what we think or see is being conveyed by the patient with respect to his feelings and attitudes.

Clarifying through Summary

In one interview alone, each of the tactics of clarification mentioned thus far may be used several times in addition to other communication skills. As we grow in our ability to clarify through these various tactical approaches, we need another means of clarification, called summarization, through which we consolidate and review the information we have obtained.

Summarization is a capsule review of the content and feelings discussed during an interview. It is given clearly so that the patient can see what progress has been made, giving him a chance to see his contributions and to determine whether they have been pertinent and helpful. Summarization also gives him one final opportunity to correct any of the information being reviewed.

Summaries signal the conclusion of the period of time agreed upon between ourselves and a patient for an interview, and they usually are offered during the last ten minutes, at which time patients are not encouraged to bring up new topics. They allow time not only for review, but also for patients to begin adjusting to the end of the interview. Just as summaries give evidence of progress, they also give evidence of the areas needing development during future interviews. The material from these areas can be used to assess the present interview and plan the next one. In summarizing progress, patients have a clearer understanding of the direction they are taking during succeeding interviews.

As Richardson observes, summaries can be used to end a particular conversational line within the interview, they can be used at the end of the interview, and they can be used when a series of interviews within the helping relationship have concluded. In addition, they can be used to begin an interview, especially if several days or weeks have elapsed since the last one [13]. Opportunities for summarizing progress with our patients should not be overlooked, because it is through summary that the patient's role of participant in the helping relationship is reaffirmed.

Whatever tactic we use to improve our ability to clarify, it must be used to promote mutual understanding between ourselves and our patients. These tactics, when used consistently, protect us from making unwarranted and unfounded assumptions about them. If one cardinal guideline emerges from this discussion of tactics in clarification, it is never to assume. Assumptions result from laziness or unwillingness to check the facts. Making an assumption, for example, can lead to the administration of Demerol, when clarification may have indicated that only Empirin compound was required.

An important way we can come to understand what our patients mean is through clarification, just as we must provide them with the means of understanding us. However and wherever we use the various tactics of clarification, their collective purpose can be stated simply: "What clarifies — verifies."

COMMUNICATING SUPPORT

Interviews are not made up entirely of questions and answers. They, together with silence, set into motion patterns of thought, which continue the course of an interview. To many patients, the motion perpetuated by these particular skills is not enough to convey the support, empathy, and understanding they may need. In the haste to procure data, we often underestimate the use and value of less apparent acts of communication, which are as essential in the support of patients as are the more obvious techniques we may employ. The way in which we respond nonverbally to a patient and the willingness to listen and to make ourselves available to him all begin the process of communicating our wish to help, understand, and share whatever may concern him. Every day our encounters with patients provide us with many opportunities to extend some kindness, some gesture of compassion and empathy. A comforting glance, a smile, a touch, enjoyment of the fragrance of flowers, and pleasure from an amusing story or cartoon all play a part in extending to a patient the unspoken invitation to use us for support during times of stress or need.

These efforts may require a more tangible form — some word or phrase that simply states our concern and our willingness to help. Simple statements do this in a way questions cannot. They do not demand or interrogate as questions may appear to do; instead, they respond to a need and invite participation between ourselves and patients. Such is its task — the invitation to communicate.

The process of communicating verbal support (that is, the verbal invitation to communicate) is comprised of several steps. First, we become aware of a change in behavior or perhaps in the tone of our patient's voice during our encounters with him. These changes may be overt, or almost imperceptible, but they are deviations from his previous behavior. Second, whatever is being conveyed by him in this manner is being expressed with difficulty or is contrary to his usual mode of expression. Third, in recognizing that he needs to express his thoughts and concerns, we initiate verbal action by commenting on his difficulty. However individualistically we convey our support, empathy, and understanding to patients, one common message unites our intent with our patients' need — that we want to help them, that we see what they are going through, and that it is hard to achieve alone.

The conditions of support are present in every helping relationship, but recognition is necessary to initiate assistance for them. Every day there are many instances in which our patients are not aware of or cannot easily convey their need for support. Without recognition, patients' needs become less evident, and opportunities to provide support become less obvious to us. Think of it another way. Support is similar to a piece of wearing apparel — a blouse or a shirt. The collar, buttons, cuffs, pockets, and style all point to the function of it — to be put on and worn. No piece of clothing has value if it is not *picked up and worn*. People in need are analogous. Their feelings, the cues they convey, and the stresses experienced because of their particular situations are like the parts of the shirt or blouse; they are all waiting to be picked up and used in some way that will assist them with self-expression and emotional comfort. Our task is to recognize these items (or cues), try them on for size, and give voice to what we see or feel with respect to our patient's needs. Initiating supportive communication conveys our willingness to help and to be available when that help is needed, and the effort is not missed by our patients.

Communicating support does not guarantee magical solutions; it is not meant to do so. We do not have all the answers, and most of us realize that in time, but in various situations we are expected to have them. The pressure to do is very real, and many of us grow very uncomfortable with the prospect that *to help* means to *assist with*, and not to accomplish everything *for* the patient.

After many encounters with patients in the hospital and the community, what we do realize is the necessity to empathize with others. Empathy evolves in so many ways: being available when we are needed, being able to say a word or two that simply state we are "with" that person, trying to be aware of what he may be going through even though we may never really know, and letting him know that our answers are not pat, but that we will stay and help him find an answer. In these moments, we become that person for a fleeting instant, allowing ourselves to participate momentarily in *his* feelings and experiences. During that time we communicate, in our own unique way, that the other person is worth the effort. Such moments in a helping relationship do much to promote a patient's self-esteem; they renew, motivate, and strengthen his efforts to pursue his own goals.

Let us look at the conditions of offering support through the following situation:

> An elderly Italian man was being visited by a nursing student once a month. Since he had no relatives, he looked forward to each of her visits and expressed this to her every time she came. During one of their last visits, the nursing student brought up the topic of termination of the visits. He became quite excited and was visibly upset. He had difficulty speaking and kept repeating several phrases. "Change, change, no good. You be my friend always and make visits like you do now. You no leave — that no good. You be my friend; I be yours. Other girls come and go, but you stay!" Seeing his difficulty with the subject and his increasing anxiety, the nursing student replied during a pause, "It must be hard to see another nursing student leave again." With this remark, she noticed that the elderly gentleman became more at ease, and though he still expressed his concern, his words were more coherent.

In this example, the nursing student saw a change of behavior in the elderly Italian man. He had always looked forward to the visits and expressed his delight in seeing her. When termination of the visits was mentioned, his communication behavior altered. His words were short and his sentences incomplete, and he was visibly upset. When he paused, the nursing student's supportive comment crystallized what he had been trying to say. With this remark, he relaxed a bit. She surmised through his verbal and nonverbal behaviors what had been hard for him to say.

Another example of supportive communication is the following situation:

> Mrs. B was admitted to a medical ward with a painful malignancy. During the following six weeks her physical condition gradually worsened. It was essential for her to maintain her activities of daily living, which included sitting in a chair and walking, so that she would not succumb to a respiratory infection. Though she was quiet by nature, and amiable,

in the past few days she adamantly refused to sit up in a chair or walk because it was painful to do so. One morning during her bath, she became short-tempered about the prospects of getting out of bed and into a chair. As the time to get out of bed drew near, she looked very tense and fearful. Noting this cue, the nurse said, "Lean on me — I'll help you all I can." While she still experienced discomfort, Mrs. B. looked less tense than she had, and she did manage to seat herself in the chair.

To be verbally supportive means to initiate actions that reaffirm the ego-integrity of our patients and other people in similar need. Sincerely offered, such comments do much to promote rapport and understanding between our-selves and patients. The availability implicit in supportive comments acts as a preface to any further communication exchanges within the interview or the helping relationship. In any event, such comments often suffice, because they may indicate to our patients that someone is participating in their health care and realizes in part what they may be experiencing and trying to share with us. Anytime we can offer verbal support, those comments, along with our nonverbal communication, serve as a visible and reflective measure of our patient's worth. Every patient needs a perimeter of support and every one of us needs to remem-ber the quality of that perimeter is something that we must deliberately help to build.

SUMMARY

Our discussion of the nurse as a source-encoder began with the differentiation of therapeutic communication and our own everyday communication. The words pivotal to understanding that difference have been identified as *plan* and *consciously influence.* We have discussed the necessity of planned communica-tion as a prerequisite to any nursing action we may take on behalf of patients, and how it enables their interests to be better served. Some of the common misunderstandings about therapeutic communication have been discussed with the hope that an awareness of them will help in our attempts to be more authen-tic with our patients.

The nursing interview continued our discussion of the communication skills necessary to professional nursing practice. An interview depends upon the communication approach presented by the nurse relative to the needs of patients. In an effort to give and receive information in an interview situation, several communication skills are potentially useful. Among them are various types of questions, silence, and tactics of clarifying and of communicating support. Depending on the purpose, level of understanding, and amount of anxiety, these skills, when used together, alternately, and with variety, enable us to facilitate more effective nurse-patient communication.

NOTES

1. Keltner, John. *Interpersonal Speech-Communication: Elements and Structures*, p. 264.
2. Ibid., p. 265.
3. A composite definition compiled by the nursing faculty of the University of San Francisco, January, 1968.
4. Keltner, op. cit. (note 1), pp. 268–269.
5. Ibid., p. 269.
6. Gorden, Raymond L. *Interviewing: Strategy, Techniques and Tactics*, pp. 206–207.
7. Richardson, Stephen A., et al. *Interviewing: Its Forms and Functions*, pp. 149–150.
8. Ibid., p. 204.
9. Gorden, op. cit. (note 6), p. 188.
10. Richardson, op. cit. (note 7), p. 204.
11. Ibid., p. 163.
12. Ibid., pp. 161–163.
13. Ibid., pp. 163–169.

BIBLIOGRAPHY

Bermosk, Loretta, and Morden, Mary Jane. *Interviewing in Nursing*, New York: Macmillan, 1964.

Bernstein, Lewis, and Dana, Richard. *Interviewing and the Health Professions.* New York: Appleton-Century-Crofts, 1970.

Burd, Shirley, and Marshall, Margaret, eds. *Some Clinical Approaches to Psychiatric Nursing.* New York: Macmillan, 1963.

Garrett, Annette. *Interviewing: Its Principles and Methods.* New York: Family Service Association of America, 1942.

Goldin, Phyllis, and Russell, Barbara. Therapeutic Communication. *American Journal of Nursing*, 69:1929, 1969.

Gorden, Raymond L. *Interviewing: Strategy, Techniques and Tactics.* Homewood, Ill.: Dorsey, 1969.

Jourard, Sidney. *The Transparent Self.* Revised ed. Princeton, N.J.: Van Nostrand, Reinhold, 1971.

Jourard, Sidney. *Disclosing Man to Himself.* Princeton, N.J.: Van Nostrand, 1969.

Kahn, Robert, and Cannell, Charles. *The Dynamics of Interviewing.* New York: Wiley, 1957.

Keltner, John W. *Interpersonal Speech-Communication: Elements and Structures.* Belmont, Calif.: Wadsworth, 1970.

Lewis, Garland K. *Nurse-Patient Communication.* Dubuque, Iowa: William C. Brown, 1969.

Lifton, Walter M. *Working with Groups*, 2nd ed. New York: Wiley, 1967.

Matson, Floyd, and Montagu, Ashley, eds. *The Human Dialogue: Perspectives on Communication.* New York: Free Press, 1967.

Muller, Theresa G. Dynamics of Communication in Nursing. *Journal of Nursing Education*, 1:9, 1962.

Pitcher, George, ed. *Wittgenstein: The Philosophical Investigations.* Garden City, N.Y.: Doubleday, 1966.

Richardson, Stephen A., Dohrenwend, Barbara S., and Klein, David. *Interviewing, Its Forms and Functions.* New York: Basic Books, 1965.

Ruesch, Jurgen. *Therapeutic Communication.* New York: Norton, 1961.

Stockwell, Martha, and Nishikawa, Herbert. The Third Hand: A Theory of Support. *Journal of Psychiatric Nursing and Mental Health Services,* May–June, 1970, p. 7.

6

Knowledge Level

ECOLOGY

Concern for the state of our environment has, in the past few years, become of increasing importance. We all have a responsibility to prevent the depletion of our natural resources and to eliminate ecological blights, including noise, overcrowding, anonymity, poverty, and other unhealthful conditions. Our obligations extend beyond the environment as such to each individual as he interacts within it and is affected by that interaction — a field called human ecology. The problems of our environment are the concern of every person, but how people are affected by those problems is the concern of professional nurses everywhere.

As citizens, we are concerned about the increasing pollutants in our air and streams; as nurses we must be concerned with their potentially hazardous effects upon health. As citizens we become alarmed by the overcrowded living conditions in the inner core of our urban areas, but as nurses we must be knowledgeable about the social calamity that can result from them. Noise, violence, fear, and high crime rates are familiar problems; as nurses, we must realize that they influence the physical and mental health of all individuals.

Case findings and statistical evidence of disease do not give a complete picture of the quality of health within the community. With increasing awareness that environmental factors can support or threaten the health on which we depend, we have begun to see the precarious balance between ourselves and our environment. For this reason we must look for and recognize the potential dangers that may alter this equilibrium. Assessment of health must include environmental factors if it is to be complete.

Health is not an absolute. Being healthy implies neither an absence of disease nor a state of perfection. The World Health Organization suggests that health is a "complete state of physical, mental and social well-being" [1]. This implies a balance — a harmony between our physical, mental, and social selves. Harmonies vary, and so do levels of health. Each individual presents his own level of health and for this reason it is a comparative term, used to describe his strength and abilities to function in relation to others.

Ruth Freeman observes that there is little agreement as to what constitutes health and suggests that it be considered in terms of what is possible as well as desirable for an individual to achieve [2]. The term *what is possible* places greater emphasis on a person's own strength, and abilities, in addition to the ability he has in resources conveying those assets to us. The person's reservoir of health and the communication of his assets are a cooperative partnership that makes the desired goal of health a possible one.

Regardless of what health may mean to us, it does not exist in a vacuum. It is determined by an environment that is both conducive and hostile to its achievement. We must begin to examine this environment in order to determine how best to help our patients to achieve a level of health that promotes and supports maximal integration of their physical, social, and mental well-being.

Early Hippocratic teachings proposed health as the expression or outcome of man's alliance with the environment; we must now examine both the physical and the social elements that comprise that environment. When people are confronted by intolerable conditions, such as impure water, out-dated and substandard housing, rat infestation, high illegitimate birthrates, and skyrocketing venereal disease rates, it is understandable that they despair, become alienated, and feel the futility of trying to cope with situations over which they believe they have no control. Their actions are guided by fear; their frustrations are released through anger and violence. Everywhere social unrest pervades individuals who are demanding more immediate improvements in their socioeconomic and their health status.

We must seek out and assist these people in achieving what is possible for them. We must come to understand them and learn about environmental influences from them. Admittedly, it is not an easy task, because many communities are clustered by nationality and divided by prejudice. Environmental problems of a community, a neighborhood, or a home may be easy enough to see, but they are not solved simply through identification. We must see the problems through the eyes of the people experiencing them. Consequently, we must be there to listen and to learn their perceptions of the difficulty and their ways of communicating them, because our perception of it may not be the same as theirs. These endeavors help us gain information and broaden the concept of environmental influences, as it did for the nursing student in the following example:

In my first few visits, I asked Mrs. R. for specific information about the condition of her home and neighborhood and how she functions within the city. I used that information to compare the ecological factors we have discussed in class that influence people in our society. I found, for example, that urban decay is a process that is very evident in Mrs. R.'s neighborhood. Many houses have chipped paint and weakening boards. There are several abandoned homes as well. Mrs. R. describes her neighborhood as "dismal," compared to what it was like forty years ago. She has a chance to move to the suburbs where her daughter lives, but she has decided to stay in her home for the present; she is used to it and can be independent. This shows her autonomy and her perception of reality; she has made a choice from her knowledge of the facts, yet she can change her decision and move if it becomes physically and economically necessary to do so. According to Mrs. R., crime, another element of poverty and urban decay, has increased since World War II, and she keeps her door locked and protected while she is home or out.

Talking with Mrs. R. about how she sees herself in relation to her environment has really opened my eyes to things I never realized — and yet over the years she has experienced them daily. I am amazed by her grit and her ability to live independently and not be totally overcome by the changes she has seen over the years. The hardest part comes next. How do I use this information that I have gathered and read about? I have been giving a lot of thought to it. Now, this whole aspect of nursing — getting involved with people (and well ones at that!) in the community — is something I had not expected to be doing in nursing. I guess I have a lot to learn. However, I have made plans about at least incorporating some of this information into our visits and hopefully helping her assess and evaluate her perceptions about this topic periodically.

Before visiting Mrs. R. again, I plan to: (1) look up recent changes (e.g., mobility, crime, and incidence of disease) in her neighborhood; (2) utilize any opportunities that may arise as a result; and (3) determine facilities that can offer help if she needs them, such as police, health department, and senior center. In my interviews I plan to ask how she gets around the city now, and whether there have been any changes in her activity patterns due to decreased physical ability. I plan to observe and listen to verbal or nonverbal indications of "mental pollution," such as fear and tension.

I am concerned about her home and its safety. I would like to investigate to what extent the inadequate heating in her house really bothers her or limits the use of her home. What does she feel about it? What can be done about it? These are just some of the ideas I have. I want to begin with them and then reassess the situation since there are not many visits left. There is much to think about in relation to Mrs. R., and she is a lady who is relatively independent and healthy. If *she* has these concerns, what more might others have who are not in such good shape!

Here we see one nursing student becoming aware of environmental influences on one life. The positive and negative influences of both the individual and the environment are illustrated in another way by a nursing student who visited an elderly couple in her community:

*Diagrammatic Presentation of the Relationship of the
Environment and Health on Mr. & Mrs. J.* [3]

Conditions varying within the host (Mr. & Mrs. J.)

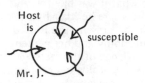

Constitution: slight build
Age: 75
Physical condition: mending
broken hip; recent eye surgery
Attitudes toward self: shy, dependent, fearful of walking, intro-
spective, responds best in a one-
to-one relationship
*Growth, development, self-actual-
ization:* grade school education,
lost interest in his hobbies, is
fond of animals

Constitution: medium build
Age: 70
Physical condition: no acute or
chronic illness
Attitudes toward self: outgoing,
autonomous, quite verbal,
enjoys groups, gets openly
annoyed
*Growth, development, self-actual-
ization:* accomplished in arts
and crafts, has college education

Conditions varying in the environment of Mr. & Mrs. J.

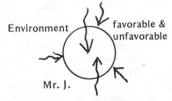
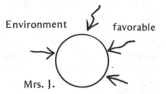

Shelter: comfortable home
Hazards: steep stairs and hills
Nutrition: poor, relies on candy
bars, sandwiches, and soda
Social patterns: solitary activities
Economic conditions: decreased
income, neighborhood old
Environmental mastery: lets community come to him; hesitant
to form new interpersonal relationships

Shelter: comfortable home
Hazards: steep stairs and hills
Nutrition: good; tries to include
the basic four
Social patterns: group activities
Economic conditions: same as
husband's
Environmental mastery: goes out
into the community; forms new
interpersonal relationships and
sustains them

In this diagram I have tried to demonstrate how I see this family in
relation to their environmental, physical, and mental well-being. Mr. and
Mrs. J. are classified in my illustration as hosts. I have classified Mrs. J.

as a host who is resistant. By this I mean a person in whom there is a balance between internal turmoils and stresses, and varieties of adaptations, knowledge, and attitudes she uses to meet them. This is not the case with Mr. J., who is, in my illustration, a susceptible host. Mr. J. is susceptible because as a person he does not appear to have the variety of personal resources necessary to adapt to various stressful situations. Therefore, he is much more inclined to be affected by adverse stresses, particularly those of an environmental nature. This does not exclude physical and mental illnesses, however. His recent physical illnesses directly affect his ability to conduct himself independently and without fear in his environment.

The resistance or susceptibility of the J. family as hosts is closely intertwined with their environment, which includes their home, their neighborhood, and the community in which they are residing. One's environment is considered favorable when it can withstand the impacts made upon it by various environmental agents, such as noise, urban decay, physical safety, and overcrowding. The opposite is true when the environment is considered unfavorable.

Again the differences in the J. family become apparent in the diagram. Mrs. J. moves with ease in her environment and is able to cope satisfactorily with various stresses from within the environment. Mr. J., however, is more cautious. Because of his recent broken hip he has limited his environmental domain to his home. Even there he is cautious. His faulty vision and his fear of hip re-injury have caused him to perceive his environment (i.e., his home) as unfavorable.

The status of the J. family as hosts and their perceptions of their environment also play a part in the determination of their positive mental health. Several factors are involved in the assessment of positive mental health. They are: (1) attitude toward one's self; (2) style and degree of growth and development or self-actualization; (3) integration; (4) ability to exert autonomy; (5) perception of reality; and (6) environmental mastery [4]. Gaps or disruptive factors in any one of these characteristics, together with the threats from physical illness and the environment, all play a part in determining the balance of health necessary to an individual and his family. These are particularly evident in the J. family, which I found after I began to assess them in terms of their positive mental health. To reiterate briefly the assessments made in my illustration:

Attitudes toward one's self

Mrs. J. is outgoing, friendly, and quite verbal. She thoroughly enjoys participating in group situations and does not hesitate to assume a leadership role when called upon. Mr. J. is aware of his health status and is not given to active socialization — even with a group in his own home. At these times Mrs. J. plays the dominant role. On a one-to-one basis this does change. When he is comfortable with another person, Mr. J. is able to share his views and gives evidence of an alert, interested mind. He does not do this except when drawn out. Mr. J. appears less sure about himself in contrast to his wife.

Style and degree of growth and development or self-actualization

Mrs. J. has received more formal education than her husband. She has won contests in arts and crafts. In addition, she was named senior citizen of the year several years ago. She can certainly look back with pride (as she has) on her achievements. Mr. J., on the other hand, has had less formal education. Since retirement he has been relatively inactive. He was interested in woodworking but has not pursued this since his eyesight has been failing. He has become very fond of animals and knows much about them. When he does talk about his old job, he does so with fondness and few regrets.

Integration

Both Mr. and Mrs. J. tolerate frustration well. She seems to get more outwardly annoyed at things, whereas he ignores them. Mr. J. does not actively combat frustration. Though he gets frustrated when he can not find anything to do around the house, he does not actively seek things to do. She, on the other hand, is always on the go and does not get bored — she does not have the time!

Autonomy

Mrs. J. is independent. She goes on trips outside the city and rides the bus to and from shopping, her senior centers, and church. She needs little or no assistance. Although Mr. J. cooks his own meals and seems to get along well when his wife is not there, I would not assess him as an autonomous person. He depends a great deal on his wife for reminders, such as when to put on a sweater, turn up the heat, answer the phone, and put on his glasses. He needs coaxing to attend social functions. His ability to make independent decisions and feel confident about them is limited.

Perception of reality

I feel Mr. J has a good perception of reality. I believe he is empathetic and sympathetic with people, perhaps even more so than his wife. I have never seen him engage in behavior that is spiteful or embarrassing to others as his wife is prone to do. In this way, he seems sensitive to others when he is with them.

Environmental mastery

As my diagram indicates, Mrs. J. goes out into the community and is able to form and sustain new interpersonal relationships during such excursions. Mr. J., however, waits for the community to come to him and does not extend himself beyond his home, with the exception of an occasional walk to the corner. He does have a dog, which means a great deal to him, but other than this he retains a certain feeling of inadequacy within his environment, which increases his perception of being overwhelmed by its demands. His ability to form new relationships is limited and dependent to a certain extent on his wife's contacts.

We now have a better picture of the physical and mental health and environmental influences of the J. family. Both Mr. and Mrs. J. should continue to maintain interaction between themselves and their environment to keep mentally and physically well. I think it is clear at this point that Mr. J. requires more nursing interventions than his wife. Supporting the positive mental health he has and finding ways he can meet some of his needs within his limited environment is one way to start. Though his eyesight is limited, it is far from being totally handicapping. Perhaps there is something he can do involving gross movements with wood. At least it is worth a try. Getting him out into the community is another approach, providing he is assured of his personal safety. Understandably he will be dependent on me to take him, but perhaps one compromise would be in letting him make the decisions about the trip in order to encourage his autonomy and a more favorable attitude of himself. Without an assessment that included the environment of this family, I would never be able to begin formulating a complete plan of nursing action.

These two examples illustrate the importance that all ecological factors, both positive and negative, have within the community.

Health settings have an ecological influence on patients because they are physical and social environments that can foster positive or negative attitudes toward health and health care. The purpose in these situations is to work cooperatively with each patient in making optimal use of his strengths and abilities. Balance and perspective are important in insuring physical, mental, social, and environmental equilibrium relative to health care. Without balance and perspective, the purpose of the care of patients becomes narrowed and distorted.

Intensive care units, for example, unwittingly provide an environment rich with opportunities for such nursing approaches. When dramatic, often heroic, efforts are being made to save a patient's life and life processes are being incessantly monitored, no consideration is given to the effect the mechanized atmosphere may be having upon the patient. Although physiological crises are abated in these settings, many psychological crises occur as a result of the intense pace of this electric environment.

Very early in the postoperative period, kidney and heart transplant patients not only succumb emotionally to the isolation they experience among so many machines, but also respond adversely to the paucity of the social environment. Mental patients put into the bland environment of state hospitals reflect their surroundings through their attitudes of listlessness. In contrast, they become animated when provided with sensory stimulation during excursions into the community. In our haste to correct the problems of illness and to secure the health of our patients, we often fail to recognize that they as *people* are also interested and involved in the kind and quality of nursing care they receive from us.

Competent nursing care implies totality of care — a totality that incorporates the environmental well-being of our patients into consistent nursing practice. Often this aspect of our practice has been compromised for expediency. We *say* that environmental factors are a part of accepted nursing practice, yet we have not gone much beyond bestowing our patients with the antiseptic tidiness they have come to expect from us over the years. Beyond this ritualistic approach, a patient's environmental comfort has a low priority among many of us who feel we have more important things to do relative to nursing care.

If totality of care is what we teach and mean to give our patients, the relationship between patients and their total (including community) environment and its effects must be germane to that care. The environmental needs of patients in the community and in specific health settings cannot be altered until we have thoroughly explored the factors that adversely influence them. This demands more of us than the passivity of helplessness or the security of intellectual awareness. Changes in our community environments and in our health settings are made by activists in nursing who daily observe and collect and assess data about the environment that may affect the health status of any human being.

The more health knowledge and care are extended into the community, the more we begin to realize how much each person's health is influenced by his environment, and what each person must contend with in order to function within it. Future nursing care will be determined by how actively all of us, students and registered nurses, work to improve the environment and the health settings in which our patients are found, and to incorporate this improvement into our total nursing care.

THE CONCEPTS OF PREVENTION

When prevention is considered, there often is a disparity between its formulation as a concept and its implementation as a nursing action. When such concepts are discussed in a classroom, they sound impressive, but because the reality of their application seems outside more traditionally oriented nursing, they are often received skeptically and considered either impractical, frivolous, or unrelated to nursing. Translating the concepts of prevention into an activity is a dilemma immediate to us in the profession of nursing.

The act of prevention requires both decision and action by deliberate efforts to stop a threat from being realized. These concepts, that is, primary, secondary, and tertiary prevention, were conceived by Dr. Gerald Caplan in order to assess the mental health status and needs of a community. In their successive perimeters Dr. Caplan saw each area of prevention building upon the other. Primary prevention is the ideal or ultimate goal, and it concerns tasks directed toward reducing the incidence of mental illness so that it does not occur. Progressively, secondary prevention involves those tasks directed to ending the mental disorder soon after it occurs; tertiary prevention is concerned with reducing the consequences of mental disorders.

The concept, as it was conceived by Dr. Caplan, is timely. The rapid pace at which we live and the convulsive changes within our social institutions force us to adapt. If we are unable, emotional problems and mental illness result. There is mounting evidence that one in ten of us succumbs to emotional dysfunction of some kind [5].

The framework provided us through the concepts of prevention is not frivolous or unrelated to the *total* experience of nursing. What makes these concepts useful and practical is their applicability to *all* people everywhere — of any age, in any circumstance, and at any level of health. Although conceived for use in the field of mental health, the concepts of prevention have extended into areas of physical, social, and environmental health.

We know, for instance, that illness is disruptive to the physical, social, and mental balance in an individual. Sometimes these disruptions result from the lack of substances basic to life, such as the lack of insulin in the diabetic patient, of mothering in an infant, or of antibody production in an infectious process. They can also result from a lack of social substances, such as a steady income.

The missing substances are needs or, as Caplan says, a shortage of life supplies [6]. In addition, disruptive factors can result from having too many supplies at any one time or over a prolonged period of time and include factors such as excessive noise, polluted air, and overcrowded living conditions. These supplies can be incorporated into our physical functioning and can involve metabolic and physiological processes. For example, excessive intake of food can result in obesity, just as excessive production of hydrochloric acid (because of increased stress) can precipitate gastric ulcers. Our responsibility is to provide, substitute for, or reduce these needs, whatever they may be, for individuals who need them, so that they can function better within the community.

Illness is a condition we can understand; its signs and symptoms are distinct, as is its treatment. The focus and activity of nursing have long been centered on problems of illness, or upon people with problems, that is, overt needs requiring highly skilled nursing and medical intervention. Even though we will continue to have patients with illness, not all people with whom we interact are ill or have problems. As prevention receives greater emphasis in nursing, we find the focus on health unsettling because we have become programmed in directing our attention to problems or illness. When there are no problems in our exposure to people, there are no roles for us to assume and no functions for us to perform according to our present understanding of nursing.

If the term *problem* must be used, why could we not begin to use it in relation to health instead? What are the problems of maintaining wellness? What do we know about how people keep well, not just in the physical sense, but socially, emotionally, and environmentally? What can be learned from these comparatively healthy people in the community that could be used to help others less able to achieve a comparable level of wellness?

Numerous factors may assist people in functioning independently within a perimeter of wellness: cultural background, a change in life style or attitude, close family ties, or perception of themselves in today's world. We can be reasonably sure that most of these people have encountered a variety of problems throughout their lives, just as we can be reasonably sure that, for the most part, they have found and used personal strength and resources in reaching solutions. Whatever the particular personal strengths and resources are, they need to be identified and described. Furthermore, the use of personal problem-solving needs not only to be supported and reinforced, but also to be promoted and nurtured in people who are less able to use it in maintaining health. This function is very important, because supplying or providing for the needs of our citizens and supporting their ego-integrity is a goal of primary prevention.

One element may help us span the gap between the *idea* of prevention and its *practice* in the community. That element is closeness. What is closeness in nursing but to be physically present in the various life spans of people? It is this presence that allows us to anticipate, identify, and replenish their life supplies *before* a problem arises or begins to be a recognized threat. Closeness means conveying to people in need that we are available to them. Closeness allows us the opportunity to discover who these people are and identify their needs and concerns. Without proximity and the information gained through it, the concepts of prevention cannot be used intelligently.

Because of its traditional use in nursing, closeness may be taken for granted or ignored, yet this role function offers us the chance to break out of more conventional nursing approaches. Think of it. If we acknowledge that nursing takes place wherever people in need are located, we cannot allow ourselves to become confined within the walls of hospitals and outpatient clinics. If we recognize that placing ourselves in close proximity to these people is the inroad to making help available for them, using the variety of settings within the community extends the element of closeness to those in need elsewhere. Recognition of these two factors (i.e., the location of people in need and the use of closeness) makes settings such as hotel lobbies, downtown libraries, department store lounge areas, local parks, city prisons, and senior centers potential nursing laboratories in which to implement the concepts of prevention.

The closeness that results from the helping encounters between nurses and patients requires time — the consistent use of it, generously given and purposefully used in settings *where that patient is located.* Into these helping proximities the nurse brings involvement, concern, trust, interest, a status of equality, and a sharing of views that promote an acceptance of the nursing functions about to be implemented. Dr. Gerald Caplan observes that the ability to reach patients in their environment, the ability to be consistently available, and the ability to share oneself with another in acceptance and trust are the characteristics of closeness that are uniquely suited to nursing [7]. The element of closeness in relation to prevention, as one concept, is being adopted by an increasing number of people in the health professions.

Our nursing efforts are one-dimensional as long as our efforts relative to closeness and prevention are directed only to members of the community who must *come to us* in the hospital. These people already have a recognized difficulty that can and must be taken care of within the hospital setting. Nursing care, under these circumstances, involves secondary and tertiary prevention because a problem (i.e., illness) has arisen that must be diagnosed and either corrected or treated so that the consequences permit a patient some means of functioning.

Nursing actions taken in these two areas of prevention are necessary, but they are taken *after the fact* — the fact of illness. No nurse can become involved in the realities of illness without having thought at least once, *"What if* we could have gotten to this patient sooner?"* or *"What* would have happened *if* this patient had known what to do or where to go?"* or *"What* would have happened *if* this patient had had someone to talk to?"* These "what if's" are just as much our concern as the efforts we make caring for the physical and emotional problems of patients in hospitals. We *have* to make them more than wishful thinking. Every day deprivations, continual stresses, loneliness, and acts of desperation take their toll on young and old alike, and each time they add another sad postscript to a well-meant but impotent effort on our part to initiate primary prevention in the community.

Applying the concepts of prevention (especially primary prevention) requires us, and this includes nursing students, to be deployed into the community. Deployment does not mean a brief exposure to community health needs just prior to graduation; it means commitment to the idea that the problems of health are as vital to our patients and our role as are the problems of illness. How will the problems of health be recognized and dealt with if there are none of us *in* the community to identify and describe them more fully? The attitudes of the public toward health and health care are not likely to be changed unless we begin to change our circumscribed attitude and role in meeting the health needs of the community. The act of prevention permits us, as nursing students and professional nurses, to use the element of closeness in a creative, innovative way. Being *in* as well as *a part of* the community communicates our concern to and for the community in a way that few other efforts in nursing can. Committing ourselves to employing prevention in this way makes the idea more of a reality than it has been in the past.

NOTES

1. Evans, Frances M. C. *The Role of the Nurse in Community Mental Health,* p. 84.
2. Freeman, Ruth B. *Community Health Nursing Practice,* pp. 4—5.
3. Adapted from Rogers, Edward. *Human Ecology and Health,* p. 166.
4. Jahoda, Marie. *Current Concepts of Mental Health,* pp. 23—64.
5. Evans, op. cit. (note 1), p. 84.
6. Caplan, Gerald. *Principles of Preventive Psychiatry,* pp. 31—34.
7. Caplan, Gerald. *Concepts of Mental Health and Consultation: Their Application in Public Health Social Work,* p. 264.

Bircher, Andrea I. Mankind in Crisis: An Application of Clinical Process to Population — Environmental Issues. *Nursing Forum*, 11:10, 1972.
Burns, William. *Noise and Man.* Philadelphia: Lippincott, 1968.
Caplan, Gerald. *Concepts of Mental Health and Consultation: Their Application in Public Health Social Work.* Washington, D.C.: U.S. Department of Health, Education, and Welfare, 1959.
Caplan, Gerald. *Principles of Preventive Psychiatry.* New York: Basic Books, 1964.
D'Amelio, Rosalie F. An Approach to Health and Illness. *Nursing Science*, 3:186, 1965.
Dubos, René J. *Man Adapting.* New Haven: Yale University Press, 1965.
Dubos, René J. *So Human an Animal.* New York: Scribner, 1968.
Dunn, Halbert L. *High Level Wellness.* Arlington, Va.: R. W. Beatty, 1961.
Evans, Frances M. C. *The Role of the Nurse in Community Mental Health.* New York: Macmillan, 1968.
Freeman, Ruth B. *Community Health Nursing Practice.* Philadelphia: Saunders, 1970.
Jahoda, Marie. *Current Concepts of Mental Health.* New York: Basic Books, 1958.
Klein, Donald. *Community Dynamics and Mental Health.* New York: Wiley, 1968.
Proshansky, Harold M., Ittelson, William H., and Rivlin, Leanne G., eds. *Environmental Psychology: Man and His Physical Setting.* New York: Holt, Rinehart and Winston, 1970.
Rogers, Edward. *Human Ecology and Health.* New York: Macmillan, 1960.
Ryan, William, ed. *Distress in the City.* Cleveland: Press of Case Western Reserve University, 1969.
Theodorson, George A., ed. *Studies in Human Ecology.* Evanston, Ill.: Row, Peterson, 1961.
Toynbee, Arnold J. Man and His Settlements: An Historical Approach. *Ekistics*, 21:75, 1966.
White, Lyn, Jr. The Historical Roots of Our Ecologic Crisis. *Science*, 155:1203, 1967.

7

Attitudes

AS WE DEVELOP from childhood, we are molded and remolded by the world, its events, its people, and their ways of thinking. Our learning begins with our parents. Through their influence, our feelings, opinions, and perceptions of the world take shape unquestioningly and unthinkingly. As our spectrum of experiences increases, we unconsciously absorb additional philosophies, social expectations, and traditions. Through learning, we then may modify or reinforce our feelings and perceptions.

It is our observable and consistent behavior toward others that gives our attitudes definition; they constitute the core of our make-up as human beings, and as such are reflected in our likes and dislikes — our opinions about issues, ideas, people, and events. What we are, we are because of our attitudes, and we react instinctively to protect them when objects and people threaten the security we derive from them. Since attitudes are introduced early in our lives, and we are generally unaware of how we acquire them, we do not become aware of them until they are challenged. We continue unwittingly to assimilate them throughout our lives.

In nursing, we are concerned about all factors that affect our relationships with patients. They come from different backgrounds, nationalities, and religions and have attitudes that developed in much the same way as ours. During our interactions with them, we soon discover that nothing is communicated as quickly or as surely as our attitudes. They affect how and what we communicate; they affect the transmission of our knowledge and they clearly imply the influence of our cultural heritage.

Our attitudes are so subtle that they often convey the opposite of our original intent. At times, no degree of proficiency in conducting an interview can mask or eliminate them and their effect on patients. Because they are more instinctive than reasoned, we are not alert to the extent of their influence on us. Contact with patients who hold opposing beliefs and attitudes can shake our confidence in our ability to relate to others.

ATTITUDES: THEIR IMPORTANCE AND FUNCTION

Our attitudes are like unfolded road maps; each section of the road is marked — each bend and curve in the road charts the way we have come as it does the road yet to be traveled. In order to reach our destination, we must know where the markers are and how they will affect the journey ahead. Without these markers our journey may be hazardous.

The practice of nursing resembles such a road map because it is often a road full of markers, bends, and curves that not all of us are fully aware of or have tested. What we have instinctively absorbed and followed through a lifetime of experiences must now be identified and examined because our influence upon patients and their health care is exerted through our attitudes. Not all of them are helpful, and we are not always aware of how they may affect patients. Our growth as professional nurses comes as we identify and examine them and their subsequent influence upon patients. Without such exposure, we become less inclined to investigate and to change what has been a familiar path of behavior.

We know that attitudes are absorbed from our social environment and are accepted uncritically. In nursing, however, this can lead to interpersonal difficulties with our patients, which are communicated subtly and with impact.

Attitudes tell our patients something about ourselves. They guard our self-esteem, convey our likes and dislikes, and at the same time safeguard us from the glare of our faults and shortcomings. They tell others how we feel, and what we believe, and give expression to our basic values.

Attitudes help us adjust to the complex demands of our environment by making them seem more attractive and rewarding. These intricacies are organized and simplified by our attitudes so that we can better understand our environment and be less overwhelmed by it. In turn, our adjustment to the world improves as does our ability to relate to and get along with others. The attitudes we convey with people, as Triandis observes, improve our relationships with them because of the amount of predictability available to us.

> We have an established repertory of reactions to a given category of attitude objects. Once a social object has been classified in that category, we can employ our existing repertory of reactions. This saves us from deciding again, starting from first principles, what our reaction should be to a particular attitude object. To the extent that our system works, it

adds predictability to the events of our social environment. If we have classified the attitude object correctly and the object behaves the way similar objects have behaved in the past, we can employ our previous experience as a guide and usually be correct about the outcome [1].

We and our patients engage each other with a "repertory of reactions." Although this is an economic measure that spares us the emotional expense of continually having to make decisions about each person we meet, it can also serve as an excuse for making a decision. When it comes to caring for patients, the danger from the use of such a repertory is in conveying what we feel about people *like him*, but not *about him* as an individual. Similarly, a patient meets *us* for the first time and conveys his expectations of nurses in general, but not of us as individuals who also *happen* to be nurses. These views may be positive or negative, depending on the conditions of attitudinal learning in the past.

The predictability factors in our attitudes may result in communicating reactions that conflict with our perceptions and in misunderstanding of intent, which may have an adverse effect on our ability to relate to and care for patients. Reconciliation of these attitudinal differences and misunderstandings must begin internally and must involve exploring *what* attitudes we actually do hold and *how* they help or hinder our relationships with patients and the care involved.

ATTITUDES THAT FACILITATE COMMUNICATION IN HELPING RELATIONSHIPS

As professional nurses of whom patients have expectations, we can develop several attitudes that have a positive influence on them during interviews. They can be learned providing we are open to learning and to evaluating ourselves relative to their use. Generally, a positive attitude demonstrates our interest in patients despite the ways they present themselves to us. It reflects the confidence we have in ourselves and in our ability to relate to others. It means self-confidence that conveys a willingness to share ourselves in the exercise of responsibility to a patient and his care. A positive attitude reflects purpose — not just in the use of techniques or skills, but also in the direction we plan on behalf of patients.

Cultivating and reflecting positive attitudes as an ongoing task throughout our professional lives is not easy because so much of what we are and feel has not been open to examination before, but this should not dissuade us from the attempt. Positive and helping attitudes, such as investment, acceptance, and objectivity, can favorably influence patients and their care and compliment their identities as unique human beings.

THE ATTITUDE OF INVESTMENT

The attitude of investment is the act of deciding to give of ourselves to others. Ideally, it is employed consciously prior to the implementation of nursing care. This seems to be a natural conclusion, because it is difficult to conceive of any attitude other than of investment in our interactions with patients. Since attitudes are unconsciously culled from our life experiences, we can understand with what ease nursing activities can be implemented without realization of what nursing and patients demand of us.

The formation of our own attitude of investment in the care of patients requires a decision committing ourselves to a course of action, one which draws on our skill, compassion, and intellect in order to activate and maintain our commitment to patients. Any decision involves choice, which implies freedom with responsibility in the execution of that choice. The choice of investing ourselves in our patients is always present in nursing. We may choose to knowingly and willingly place our own resources at a patient's disposal or we may choose to function without such an investment. Whatever the decision, we begin the formation of patterns that will chart the course of our professional lives.

Investment also requires giving — giving of our feelings, attitudes, skill and knowledge whenever they are needed. Giving suggests purpose — an awareness that should preface its enactment. It is this attitude which must be present before other helping attitudes become operational, because it is our receptivity and willingness which allows investment to take root, grow, and blossom in our interpersonal relationships with patients.

The act of giving, as the precursor of helping attitudes, implies risk. Our investment in another human being is speculative at best — nothing is assured simply because we have invested our personal and professional selves. In doing so we discover that we may be investing infinitely more in our patients than we can ever hope to have reciprocated. This is the risk of investment — an unequal return on an initial offer of ourselves to patients.

For some of us, our investment is sizable. The nursing skills and the compassion for another's suffering during a terminal illness, for example, drain us of psychic energy and often exhaust our knowledge about that patient and his illness. Still we continue, willing to undergo similar experiences in order to sustain the strength and courage of someone who relies on the investment we have made. For some of us such an investment may not be possible or fully realized. The security resulting from the performance of technical skills is too gratifying and immediate to be sacrificed for the untried areas of interpersonal abilities.

It is hard to give of ourselves fully to our patients, just as it is hard to know *what* it is we are to give. In a very real sense, we come to our patients untried and unchallenged in the values, beliefs, and philosophies of living and being among people. Interactions with patients provide us with a range of situations and experiences that helps us identify not only the resources we possess, but also the extent to which we possess them and can give them to others. Each encounter with a patient mirrors to him more clearly who we are.

In turn, each encounter should also reveal to us a little more of "what we are about" in nursing — that is, do we *believe* in what we are trying to accomplish for our patient? Do we *convey* that belief to our patients, not only in the application of scientific and technical skills, but also *genuinely* in the way we *present ourselves*? Does each encounter with patients crystallize our beliefs and ideas about the way we consciously wish to practice nursing? Do we *have* a belief or idea about what the practice of nursing is for us?

Only through openness to experiences in nursing can we give definition to ourselves as invested practitioners of nursing and gain personal growth. This openness implies risk, but the hope and satisfaction beyond that risk make the act of giving — of willing and committed giving — a prevailing attitude that is genuinely communicated to our patients.

THE ATTITUDE OF ACCEPTANCE

To accept another human being. To welcome him as the living outcome of all past experiences, attitudes, and feelings. A product of life, not always positive, endearing or self-enriching, but a life ultimately *his own*. We may not totally understand his way of thinking, his way of communicating, or his reactions to other human beings, but that is not as important as remembering what he is *now*. To accept means to receive willingly the hopes, sorrows, frustrations, and mistakes he offers us. In return, we affirm through our communication his special one-of-a-kind self — different from others in the expression of his behavior, but similar in that his feelings, hopes, and dreams form a unifying bond with other human beings.

The plea to be unique yet the same as others is common to all human beings. It is more important to our patients, who are being assaulted by the stresses of illness and other equally demanding problems. Illness separates an individual from others, forces him into the role of patient, determines his future, irrespective of his needs. Such an experience influences his attitude toward himself; it becomes more negative. Differences make him feel alienated. "I am different" may mean during these stresses, "I have little or no redeeming value in relation to other people." Such feelings are demoralizing.

Acceptance of others begins with self-acceptance because we cannot accept imperfections and qualities in others until we have admitted to similar characteristics in ourselves. This is not achieved in isolation. The capacity to be open to and aware of various people and experiences contributes to self-acceptance. Such openness gives us an opportunity to absorb, continually adjust to, and change our perceptions about people and events. As this process continues, we become less intimidated by new situations and individual differences.

Security and confidence in our relationships with others comes through *what* we have learned about ourselves and *how* we came to learn it from involvement with people in the past. Self-acceptance comes from being *treated* as a worthwhile, successful, and likeable human being. To *experience* such acceptance and from it to learn to like ourselves is a cornerstone to the acceptance of others, because we cannot give to others what we do not possess ourselves.

Because self-acceptance is a continuing process, we bring to nursing a partially developed appraisal of ourselves. Through nursing practice our exposure to patients of diverse backgrounds, attitudes, and cultures continue to fire the experiential process begun in our childhood. Together with stresses and conditions of every description, we forge an increasingly realistic appraisal of ourselves. What strengths we have help us to act intelligently and dependably; our suspected shortcomings become more discernible and perhaps more understandable as we extend this awareness to our patients. In doing so, we come closer to and more comfortable in allowing patients to be what they *are*, while we assist them in achieving what they *can be*.

Such actions can lessen our tendency to judge, because we are not forced to demand that our patients be what they are not. This sounds infinitely simpler than it is, because in nursing, the patience we must exercise presumes more time than we have or are willing to use. Here again, the predictable repertory of reactions is an expedient means of assessing instant judgments about our patients. It can be hazardous, however, because as Combs points out, "disillusionment and despair in human relationships are the product of inaccurate assessments of what people are like and what can be expected of them" [2].

Insisting that people become someone other than who they are, and condemning them for this supposed inability, is an attitude that blocks acceptance of them and inhibits the flow of their communication with us. Being judgmental strongly indicates dominance over another human being, and serves as instinctive bait, continually tempting us because of the smugness of superiority it momentarily brings us. Whether or not we like it, our most difficult task is admitting to ourselves that we are, by nature, judgmental people. It is a myth to suppose we can ever totally eliminate it in ourselves, but recognizing it may be a beginning in lessening its effect upon our patients. Because of its instinctual surge during our contacts with patients, the task of neutrality is not made easier. Often our awareness in this area comes *after* we have spoken with a patient.

Allowing a patient to develop *his* thinking and decision-making in *his* own way requires a great deal of restraint and patience on our part. To interfere through judgmental pronouncements prevents the openness necessary to his experiential development. We inhibit his growth by implying he is unworthy and subtly force him to apologize to us for failing to meet *our* standards.

We may be startled by many things a patient may tell us, or disgusted, or angered, but regardless of the feelings evoked in us, we must learn and remind ourselves to view what has been shared with us in the light of the patient's experience rather than our own. This is a thankless task and a slow one, but it is necessary to the process of *learning* to accept our patients for the individuals they are.

To make acceptance a living current — something energized and exchanged between ourselves and patients — requires an atmosphere in which that attitude is possible. A patient learns to trust himself, his ideas, and his opinions when he is given the opportunity to express them without condemnation. During these moments, he can examine the substance of those ideas and opinions; it then becomes possible for him to appraise them critically and perhaps to discover constructive alternatives.

Illness poses a threat, and its appearance in any person can disturb his perceptions. Such a threat diminishes his confidence and his ability to deal with it. His need for acceptance becomes all the more apparent and is expressed in his behaviors. It is in the act of sharing these behaviors, however slight or momentary, that one attempts to communicate acceptance. In every act of trying to be accepting, we become more open — aware — energized to the experience of our patient. Whatever he shares with us is his, *not ours,* and it is what *he* shares that fosters a sense of his specialness, together with his inherent plea to respect his individuality. This is what we must nurture.

Encouraging a patient to enter into partnership with us in effecting his recovery fosters a sense of belonging in him. Without partnership there can be no involvement and no learning, and the atmosphere for acceptance diminishes. Each contact with a patient offers a variety of opportunities for cultivating a sense of belonging. The way we encourage and answer a patient's questions, the way we listen to his complaints, his fears, his opinions, and the willingness to be available to him all communicate our attempts to be open to him as an individual. Each time we fail in these attempts we say in effect that sameness — not individuality — should be his ultimate goal. This inhibits a patient's need to explore and learn from the events and people involved in his care.

Even though we learn to recognize our patients' needs for acceptance — even though we learn how the attitude of acceptance develops and influences others — even though we are aware of its implications for nursing, acceptance remains a very personal act of communication between ourselves and patients. What we accept — whom we accept — how we accept requires more than making a professional gesture and calling it acceptance. Can each of us *really* accept another person who in the circumstances of illness becomes our patient? Can we *really* accept another human being whose ideas, dress, speech, and behavior deviates even slightly from our own? Can we? That is a question for which most of us have no answer, because it implies knowing what acceptance is and having practiced it throughout our lives. For most of us, however, the answer is some-where in *each* experience we share with a patient and the way we share it *with* him. It comes each time we ask ourselves, "Can we?" When that happens, mark it well, for what we discover about acceptance along the road map labeled "me" is not how far we have come, but how much further we must go.

THE ATTITUDE OF OBJECTIVITY

Trying to develop an attitude of objectivity with patients often resembles trying to satisfy two masters. On the one hand, we are expected to invest our-selves, to be compassionate and caring in our interactions with patients, and on the other hand, we are expected to be detached and objective and to apply scientific principles to them and their care. The result is confusion as we try to convey what *seems* to be contradictory attitudes of patient care. To those of us convinced that a warm, compassionate approach is the only humane way to interact with patients, an objective or detached approach seems unfeeling and uncaring. Others of us, however, feel that anything *but* an objective, dispassion-ate approach to patients means not only overinvolvement with them, but also ineffectual nursing care.

The study of human behavior is an imprecise science. We cannot study and learn about people in as detached a manner as we can study other sciences, such as chemistry and microbiology. The reason should not be a surprise; as Pogo observed, "We have met the enemy and they are us." Our facts about human beings and their behavior are often obscured by our biases, feelings, and values. They cannot be dismissed in our search for objectivity, however, since in inter-action with others, we act on them, perceive by them, and judge by them. We must therefore *learn about* them, *learn* to live *with* them, and *learn* to *use* them discriminately. Developing an attitude of objectivity can help us achieve this.

Attempts to define objectivity reveal the recurrence of certain words and phrases, including self-discipline, evaluation, freedom from bias, practicality, restraint, emotional control, detachment, and vigilance. Using the theme derived from these words, let us define objectivity as the deliberate intellectual maneuver used to discipline and modify our emotional reactions in order to *fully* concentrate upon and realistically appraise the patient, *his* feelings, and *his* predicament.

Learning to be objective about a patient does not mean denying our feelings and emotions, but rather concentrating on his. When we are told we are not being objective, we are being informed that we have failed to put the patients' needs and feelings before our own.

Objectivity is rooted in reality; it tempers our feelings and reactions with facts and knowledge. Being objective does not mean being devoid of feelings and genuine emotion, but it does mean attaching an intellectual component (such as appraisal, knowledge, or evaluation) to them in order to understand consciously the patient's situation and our experiences with him. In other words, "one's own hopes, fears and ideas of what *should be* are set aside in favor of discovering what *is* . . . those of us working in the [helping professions] must strive to maintain vigilance over [our] own emotions and sentiments in order to . . . prevent conclusions from leaping along inviting lines of intuitive conviction and thus out distancing disciplined observation and systematic thinking" [3].

Though it is never simple to achieve objectivity, there are means by which an attitude of objectivity can be fostered. Each offers an opportunity to examine systematically a patient's situation as it pertains to his problem or need and his communication of it. In so doing, we blend our subjective perceptions with our intellectual abilities.

Problem-solving is one means of helping to achieve objectivity. The sequence of this process, namely, identification (of a patient need), description, analysis, formulation, implementation, and evaluation, offers a systematic method of uniting our intuitive and our scientific abilities. Each step offers us an opportunity to compare what we *feel* to be so with what *is* so. For example:

Identification
   What is going on here?
   What am I seeing?
   What did I hear?
   Why do I think the patient has a need or problem?
   Why does the patient think he has a need or problem?
   Did something happen?
Description
   What is the patient's background?
   Did I clarify what I saw or heard?
   Do I have the correct sequence of events?
   What did I do to facilitate getting the necessary information?
   What are my attitudes at this point?
Analysis
   What themes emerge from what I have collected?
   How does the patient view his problem?
   How does what I collected relate to the scientific knowledge I have
      learned?
   Is there anything missing from these data?
   Are any different behaviors I have observed related to the same problem?
   What cultural concepts are involved that may relate to the patient's
      needs or problem?
Formulation
   What is the best plan of action based on my observations and analysis?
   Do I have alternatives? Do they include cultural components and
      attitudes?

How do I plan to facilitate my communication approach in accordance
with my plan?
Should I test my ideas with my co-workers or instructor?
Has this method of testing revealed any gaps in my plan?
Implementation
What observations of the patient have I noted during this time?
What is going on within me?
Am I adjusting my approach to the patient's need?
Am I putting into action the plan I have formulated?
Evaluation
Did my plan accomplish what I hoped to achieve?
If so, what factors contributed to its success?
If not, what factors prevented success?
What do I need to do in order to improve?
What did I learn as a result of this plan of action?

These sample questions can be used to help in the development of systematic, objective thinking, which is essential in nursing practice.

Another method of appraisal, although not as formal as problem-solving, can also be of assistance in the examination of our communication process with patients. It also involves asking questions:

"WHO said so?"
"WHAT did he say?"
"What did he MEAN?"
"HOW does he know?" [4]

Let us look at each question more closely.

In our attempts to determine the communication origin (that is, *who*), it is essential that we clarify ambiguous terms that suggest a source. Terms such as *they, them* and *a reliable source* are not only misleading, but they also stimulate our emotions, which we are attempting to discipline and modify in nursing practice. This applies to our communication not only with patients, but with co-workers as well. One small, explainable incident can easily become distorted and magnified by use of ambiguous or exaggerated terms to elicit our sympathy or provoke our reactions. Discovering the source helps reduce margins for error.

Once we have established the origin of a communication exchange or incident, our next task is to determine as specifically as we can *what* the actual exchange was. Again, the acceptance of hearsay, or what another person may *think* was said, is not an accurate representation. Speculation or hearsay undergoes a subjective metamorphosis before it is routed to us. In all likelihood, the content of the message is altered, and if we accept it as correct, our ability to objectively appraise a situation is impaired.

Our patients' communication is rarely interpreted accurately, because there are too many ways one message can be translated and too many individual perceptions. To ensure accuracy of information, everything that is not clear to us must *become* clear if we are to attain objectivity. This requires verifying what we *feel* to be the meaning of the message with an intellectual tool, namely, clarification. Then we will be sure that the patient's meaning is communicated to us accurately.

Another means of questioning and exploring the communication we receive from patients and their families is by determining how they acquired the experiences or information. For example, if a patient saw his roommate fall out of bed and reported it to us, the source of his information was direct observation. Another patient may be knowledgeable about his illness. The source of his information may well be his doctor, or he may be in a health profession. Confusion in a family regarding the health care of one of its members may be the result of receiving different opinions from outside sources, such as friends or relatives. Discovering the level of information patients and families have as well as the sources can help us appraise and plan our communication approaches.

Every method of appraisal serves as a bridge between our subjective perceptions and our intellect. An attitude of objectivity is such a bridge — spanning the troubled waters in which a patient or his family may find themselves. The troubled waters are like currents, full of conflicting problems, pulling and battering at the people caught in them. Our first instinct is to jump in and help these people despite the bridge nearby. But what then? If we plunge into the water, we run the risk of getting caught in the current. We may not know how to swim and thus may be unable to see or reach either bank. Though we are sincere in motive, our ability to be of real help is quickly rendered ineffective.

On the other hand, knowing the water is turbulent and our ability to swim is limited, we can choose to walk on the bridge. From that perspective, the water's turbulence can be confirmed and both banks are in clear view. We can formulate and implement plans that will insure the safety of the swimmers. We are in a position to effect a rescue and to concentrate on ways to help the swimmers rather than being preoccupied with keeping ourselves afloat. Bridges are built to be crossed — to guide us over terrain that may be harmful, turbulent, untested, or difficult to cross. They were built to be used — not as an afterthought, but consistently — not by one person, but by many people.

An attitude of objectivity should be developed and used consistently as a bridge to more effective nursing practice — not as a postscript to it. It should be developed and tested with our co-workers, instructors, or both, because the perceptions and feedback received from them can assist us in increasing the validity of our perceptions and applying them to a method of systematic thinking. In doing so, an objective attitude is strengthened.

ATTITUDES THAT INHIBIT COMMUNICATION IN HELPING RELATIONSHIPS

Attitudes can have an adverse influence upon our patients, thereby inhibiting the helping intent of our interactions. They are referred to as negative attitudes because, intentionally or not, they indicate disapproval to our patients. What makes them so patently negative is that they are communicated through our nonverbal behavior, which is not as conscious, intentional, or controlable as is our verbal exchange. Negative attitudes are an immediate concern for us because they stem from two very real problems we have in learning to interview effectively: the *lack of desire* to obtain the needed information, and the doubt of our *ability* to get it [5]. Both inject a dissonant tone into our interviews with patients, and both can be misperceived and misinterpreted.

A lack of interest in achieving necessary information may stem from a dislike of our patient, a dislike of what we have to do, or a feeling that the questions are probing and therefore unsuitable for use in interviews. Whatever the reason for our feelings, we convey them through our communication skills during an interview. For instance, we may presume what a patient's response will be, and this may block out the actual response. As a result, our attempt to achieve information is incomplete and we therefore fail to pursue the depth possible in an interview and to detect the nuances in our patient's behavior.

Each new experience in nursing, such as interviewing, produces a new set of self-doubts, which plague us and cause us to question our ability to function effectively in that situation. Practice makes the newness of the experience less of a threat to us, but until we have had a good deal of practice and confidence is achieved, the level of our anxiety determines how and what we communicate with patients. Our anxiety over our ability to communicate effectively is presented to them as an embarrassed apology; in a sense, we are requesting permission and pardon for the questions.

This uncertainty and self-effacement raises more doubt in patients than is warranted in helping relationships. They are quick to detect these traits, and they begin to entertain their own doubts — doubts about our abilities, the receipt of our comfort and support, or the sincerity of our interest. These can be perceived as ego threats, which then must be defended against by additional ego-protecting behaviors. A patient who is on guard in response to such attitudes is not being assisted in a manner that facilitates a helping relationship or that supports and complements his ego-integrity.

Although negative attitudes originate within us, they are expressed in behaviors directed to others during our encounters with them. These perceptions and feelings may have nothing to do with the exchange of communication, but are based upon our perceptions about the personality and image of that individual. The recognition of how these attitudes are indirectly expressed (i.e., through our behavior) to our patients may help us to become not only more aware of what we are doing, but also better able to control them in our professional relationships.

CONDESCENSION: SEPARATE AND UNEQUAL

Even though nursing provides an opportunity to meet people from a variety of cultures, backgrounds, and religions, we often are unable to be as accepting as we might wish. Whatever the reason, we find that we dislike, disapprove of, or are apathetic toward our patients. This presents an internal and often unconscious conflict because we are also aware that a negative attitude is a deterrent to the helpfulness we try to facilitate through our communication. The compromise we demonstrate through our behavior then is an air of condescension.

Whether conveyed in manner or in tone of voice, an attitude of condescension explicitly suggests one person's superiority over another. To divorce ourselves from involvement or from the emotionalism that negative feelings may arouse, we separate ourselves from the person, suggesting that he is not as capable as we consider ourselves to be. We conduct ourselves as if every encounter with him is an act of intellectual martyrdom.

This is particularly awkward in nursing, because the roles assumed by us and by patients foster it. A nurse helps others and must have the special ability and knowledge expected of that role, whereas a patient needs help, and because of his illness is helpless, or without the special knowledge and ability to care for himself. If our role of helper is supported by an attitude of superiority, which stems from our negative feelings about a patient as a person, he is not as likely to believe that we are sincerely interested in his needs and welfare.

DIMINISHED CONCENTRATION: THE COST OF FORGETTING

The inability to concentrate on what a patient is saying indirectly expresses our lack of interest in him. Forgetting parts of a conversation with a patient, forgetting that certain questions have already been asked, and not picking up overt cues are several ways this attitude can be depicted during an interview.

As we become involved in therapeutic communication, it is not uncommon to find it difficult to concentrate on the patient and what he is saying. The day may have been a hard one for us, draining the psychic energies we would normally be using for concentration; we may be tired or in a hurry. We may have difficulty remembering conversations at all, or we may be too busy planning our next approach. Occasionally, these lapses are understandable and forgiveable, but not if they occur frequently or in response to a particular patient or type of patient.

The information a patient shares with us is often important from his point of view even though it may not be significant in relation to a particular problem.

Nevertheless, its importance to the patient should be the overriding consideration. Sharing information of any kind may be difficult for a patient, and when we establish a pattern of lapses in concentration, we increase the vulnerability a patient may be experiencing. Our attention provides him with a sense of security and protection for his disclosures, and when it is lacking, he feels exposed.

Clarification at this point is essential to the accuracy of the information we receive, but when it is overused, it can easily create the impression of forgetfulness. One solution may be to give a patient recognition by reiterating what he said earlier, thereby demonstrating that we have been concentrating on his efforts to share his thoughts and feelings with us.

LACK OF SPONTANEITY: ITS OBVIOUS ABSENCE

Being cautious and formal during interviews with patients is usually the act of a novice in search of self-confidence and security. To persist in conveying these attitudes after a reasonable amount of practice, however, can negate our efforts to build confidence. A lack of spontaneity denotes reluctance to share and exchange something of ourselves with patients. It is self-serving, because it serves our need to protect the part of ourselves that we feel we cannot expose to others. It is a confining attitude as well, because it helps us retain the sense of status we have achieved in nursing. The retention of status coupled with a cautious, formal approach to patients offers many of us a feeling of safety, since the fewer our attempts to encourage spontaneity, the fewer opportunities we provide for criticism of our efforts.

Yet basic to any helping relationship is the patient's right to be encouraged and responded to, and these cannot always be accomplished with cautious or stoically formal nods of the head. Often during periods of anxiety, when a patient's ability to perceive is already limited, such actions are unperceived. He may need something much more perceivable and visible. The absence of spontaneity deprives a patient of what he may need *of us* — affirmation that we share with him the commonality of experience. Without the reassurance derived from a thoughtful, warm, and informal responsiveness, our patients may question our sincerity.

ASSESSING CATEGORIES OF ATTITUDES

In a person's repertory of reactions, feelings and attitudes are not scattered or ill-defined. Instead, they are categorized to provide us with the simplification needed to conserve our psychic energies during interpersonal relationships. This assists us in coping adequately with individual decision-making and in assessing events and people by allowing us to behave to different events and people *as if* these events and people were identical. Therefore, a remark such as "All Italians are gangsters" relieves us of having to assess every person of Italian origin on the basis of his individual background and present interpersonal relationships, even though such a process may render our original judgment false.

The value of standardization of attitudes is in helping us deal with our perceptions, particularly if they indicate impending threats of harm to ourselves or others. For example, seeing a child dart into the street while we are driving or sitting in a bus that is about to collide with a car automatically precipitates behaviors that are defensive and are intuitively enacted as soon as the threat is perceived.

Though categorizing attitudes is a developmental process, as we have discussed previously, and though it provides us with a simplified means of dealing with interpersonal complexities, it is not without drawbacks. Its major disadvantage is that, "the broader the categories, the more inaccurate they are likely to be. The more they help us, in that they allow us to simplify our problems, the more likely they are to cause us to perceive the world incorrectly" [6]. In this respect, our biases and prejudices, in the words of the writer-philosopher Ambrose Bierce, become "a vagrant opinion without visible means of support" [7].

With this in mind, we need to explore some of the common categories of attitudes that are related to our interpersonal relationships with patients and upon which our behavior and theirs is based. When such attitudes are unrecognized and unchecked in interview situations, they interfere with our perceptions of our patients and their care because we do not realize the degree of their influence on the nursing care we offer patients.

STEREOTYPES: SQUARE PEGS AND ROUND HOLES

Stereotyping other people resembles a caricature — it exaggerates them and distorts to simplicity the more complex aspects of their personalities and cultures. Such expediency in the use of our perceptions significantly affects the subsequent course of our communication with others, because our perceptions are based upon very little knowledge of or experience with them. Stereotypes, then, are the generalized and oversimplified beliefs we hold about various groups of people, which are based upon experiences too limited to be valid in interpersonal relationships.

At this point, we must exercise caution in defining stereotypes, because they have both an accurate and an inaccurate connotation. A stereotype is considered accurate when the beliefs about a group are based upon specific information, despite the lack of contact with the group. An inaccurate stereotype, on the other hand, is based upon beliefs that are nebulous and uninformed about a group of people we are not interested in and thus not motivated to learn about. For example, if we are planning a trip to France and read a good deal about the

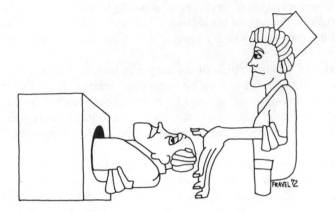

Fig. 6. Square pegs and round holes.

country, its people, and their customs, our stereotype of the French becomes
more accurate since our information has increased. This is not likely if we are
not interested in reading or studying about the French people and their culture.
Put another way, we tend to stereotype more about those we know least, and
the more we do this the less open we become to the modification of our stereotypes.

There are several ways stereotypes can perpetuate faulty assessment of others.
First, stereotypes tend to be absolute. Once a judgment has been made about a
particular trait in a group of people, all similar people are assumed to possess
that trait. Little effort goes into distinguishing this judgment or into differen-
tiating the characteristic of this group from *our own need* to see the group in
this particular stereotype. For example, an elderly patient of mid-European
origin may be vehement in her beliefs that Jewish people are devious, untrust-
worthy, and money-hungry. Because of the degree to which she holds these
beliefs, and the length of time she has held them, no amount of interaction or
information will alter her opinions, nor will she necessarily be able to understand
her motives for viewing Jewish people in this way.

Second, despite data indicating that people within a group have both similarities *and* differences, they tend to see themselves in terms of *either* their
similarities *or* their differences, but not both. Therefore the "out" group is
seen as being different from the "in" group. Mr. A., for example, belongs to a
service organization, the members of which see themselves as outgoing and
civic-minded. When another group wishes to join forces with them for a particular event, Mr. A's group tends to see this new group as being different from
themselves and quite possibly considers the new group as having nothing in
common with them.

A third factor in our assessment of others is what Triandis calls "a confusion of causes" [8]. This occurs when a specific trait is assigned to a group of people because of its racial, national, religious, or economic orientation. For example, such confusion may result in the stereotyping of Chicanos as lazy and uneducated. Let us suppose, to continue the example, that statistics substantiate lower aptitude scores among Chicanos than among whites. There may be many plausible reasons for such scores, such as previous educational background, the environment from which they came, and the environment they may be in at present. Given the same background and opportunities as whites, Chicano students may well equal or surpass them.

Last, the degree to which groups of people harbor conflict or hostility toward another group corresponds to the degree of negative stereotyping of that group. By the same token, when cooperative feelings exist between two groups, there may be positive stereotype. Student riots on college campuses, as an example, promote a great deal of negative stereotyping of students by people in the neighborhood and others who have little or no contact with student rioters. As the riots diminish and more favorable (i.e., nonviolent) behavior is exhibited, the stereotype gradually becomes more favorable. Since assessment of others requires accurate information and perception, we can see how these four factors can adversely influence the systematic collection of information needed in our interpersonal relationships.

Nothing is more predictable by its appearance in our work than are stereotypes. They pervade every aspect of our professional work and invade our attempts to identify and assess each patient's behavior on its individual merits. Because it oversimplifies our beliefs, and may be substantiated by a kernel of truth, stereotyping becomes a deceptively easy method of misguiding our nursing care.

Stereotyping of patients continues to be a strong, if not unfortunate, habit, which is supported by factors that prevent an objective assessment of our patients. Assessment of the patient as an individual comes from interaction and communication with him. These interactions can progress smoothly if we have some knowledge of the group to which he belongs. The danger here is that we may be too content with what we *think* we know of him and his group, and base our assessments of him on this superficial information. This is particularly disconcerting when a patient might be atypical of the group. Consider for a moment these examples:

> "Mr. Kelly, that Irishman, is Jewish?"
> "How can you be blond and still be Italian?"
> "You mean you're from Wisconsin and don't like beer and cheese?"

The lack of knowledge apparent in these comments reinforces the need to cling to stereotypes. When such remarks are spoken with the conviction of our beliefs, the impression of absoluteness is unmistakable, and the inclination to change is negligible. Labeling patients as good or bad represents another absolute, based upon mistaken notions of what we would like patients' behavior to be, but what, in reality, is not. Patients are, in a sense, programmed to these absolutes and become conditioned to the stereotype of "good" patient even before entering a hospital. In their minds, the alternative is not an enviable one. Basing nursing care on snap judgments and impulsive conclusions derived from fleeting impressions does very little to facilitate the sound judgments needed in such care.

The strength of any stereotype is dependent upon the degree to which our emotions are involved. We are more liable to continue reacting emotionally and coloring our perceptions if the information we send to and receive from our co-workers continues to be tinged with bias. The more we are able to listen and seek out accurate and logical information, the more we will be able to relinquish the intuitive need for stereotyping. Discouraging communication involving bias, asking for specific information about an incident or observation, helping others to do the same, and examining our feelings toward a patient can all help to eliminate perceptions that can blind our reason and cripple our effectiveness in communicating with each individual who is for a time our patient.

HALO EFFECT: THE BLINDING AURA

When we meet another person, a perceptual process is begun. We make a judgment about him based on a momentary first impression. In that instant, we classify and decide upon that person's importance to us in terms of our future relationship with him. If we decide the person is likeable, our behavior demonstrates our wish to associate with him further. If this first impression is not favorable, our behavior demonstrates our disinterest in any future association with him. Whatever the first impression, we tend to base what we think and say about that person on this initial encounter without benefit of other perceptions and information that may add to our insights of him. This is called a halo effect. Specifically, a halo effect is a judgmental perception made about another individual through which we categorize him as either good or bad on the basis of one particular characteristic, and continue to do so, even though he has other real and demonstrable personality characteristics.

By way of example, let us say that after meeting someone, we have received a good impression, possibly because that person is an avid opera fan or a history buff, enjoys movies, or is witty, articulate, or profound. Whatever the reason, we tend to continue to perceive and relate to that person in terms of what we have found pleasing, although he may have not only other good qualities, but also less endearing ones.

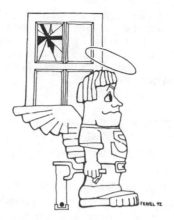

Fig. 7. Halo effect.

A halo effect can also be applied in the negative sense, that is, our initial impression may be unfavorable or bad. Although an individual may have many favorable personality traits, our behavior toward him is based upon this initial unfavorable impression. To us, he is surrounded by a glaring aura or halo, and it blinds us to his other attributes. The old proverb, "Love is blind," is a common example of a halo effect resulting from the familiarity of a close, selective interpersonal relationship.

As in most impressions, the knowledge is hastily gained, superficial, or one-dimensional. The foundations of our interpersonal relationships suffer from the paucity of richer, fuller, and more extensive perceptions of an individual. The formation of such impressions, however, and the halo effect accrued from them are inevitable because not all personality characteristics are readily observed in early phases of interpersonal relationships or clearly defined and understood by the participants. In addition, the observable characteristics may precipitate emotional reactions in others or have moral relevance to one of the participants, and therefore are not open to discussion [9]. Consider the following example:

> Miss L., aged 28, was admitted to the hospital for the removal of an ovarian cyst. Two days after surgery, she was assigned to the care of Miss C., a nursing student. Upon reading Miss L.'s medical history, Miss C. learned that she was once a prostitute. Miss L. revealed this information willingly and forthrightly, because she felt it was pertinent to her illness. The information was a shock to Miss C., who was offended by what she felt was immoral behavior on the part of Miss L., and indignant about having to take care of what she termed "that type of woman."

> Despite the fact that Miss L. was a cooperative, pleasant, articulate, and well-educated woman who had long since ceased to engage in prostitution, Miss C. continued to react to her in a brusque, disapproving manner. Miss L., puzzled by Miss C.'s attitude toward her, remarked later to her doctor, "I can't understand what's wrong. I've done nothing to offend her while I've been here."

We can see in this example how an emotional reaction to Miss L.'s earlier behavior, without prior observable and well-defined information about her as a person, generated a negative halo effect and prevented an objective and fuller assessment of the patient as an individual.

Interacting with patients and their families does not protect us from the halo effect. Stereotyping is generated from the beliefs about a *group* of people, but the halo effect results from singling people out individually on the basis of impressions formed from one personality characteristic. The halo effect, like stereotyping, leads to inaccuracy in our nursing assessments, because it fosters attitudes based on only one aspect of a patient, which are used as the basis for planning future communication and care of a patient. Such was the case in this nurse-patient interaction:

> I have been doing a lot of thinking about my second visit with Mrs. B. I am beginning to suspect a halo effect in my perception of her. Let me explain. Mrs. B. is a handsome, 82-year-old widow, whose apartment is filled with mementos of a lifetime of varied cultural interests and hobbies. She has traveled a great deal, has seen her children grow and become successful, and now can enjoy her new apartment and friends.
>
> When I met her, the first thing that came to my mind was the thought, "Now she's the epitome of a *lady.*" That impression returned on this past visit, and afterward I kept wondering why that particular quality stuck in my mind. Then it came to me. My mother had used those same words when I was smaller. My sisters and I were always told to be ladies. To my mother this meant being refined, well-mannered, gentle in our language and decorum, modest, and polite. This was her ideal for us. Being a lady means having all the qualities my mother had stressed.
>
> When I first saw Mrs. B. and her apartment, she fit the image I always thought a lady should have. Nevertheless, I should know better. Seeing Mrs. B. in that way is not really seeing her at all. I am seeing her the way I want to see her. I know intellectually she is not as perfect as I picture her. Her material comforts were not acquired magically or because she was a lady, and yet all I seem to see is the lady in her. I find myself selectively hearing what I think a lady would say, and by doing so, I feel I may be missing a great deal of information.
>
> It is strange how a seemingly insignificant thing can trigger a perception like that. I wonder how many times I have done the same thing with patients in the hospital. Right now I will have to concentrate on doing something to correct my perception of Mrs. B.

This example illustrates how one seemingly insignificant characteristic can be magnified into an aura that completely overshadows other traits and qualities. Intellectual awareness is beginning to emerge at this point, yet the nursing student realizes that it is only a partial solution. The emotional component, that is, her own reactions to the particular trait in Mrs. B., is still in operation, and until both her assessment and her evaluative abilities temper the reactive emotions, a more accurate perception is unlikely.

Any process that involves correcting the halo effect (as well as others) must be gradual, for it involves more care in obtaining information that may broaden our perceptions. In time, the impulsive judgments we make about a patient may be balanced by more accurate ones. Consistent evaluation (both by ourselves and with others) is a necessity, as it is in every nursing effort. The nursing student in the previous example is no exception:

> The halo effect remains; however, I will continue to concentrate my efforts on trying to hear that which *is said* rather than basing what I hear on the lady saying it. In my next visit, I plan to ask questions that may give me more of an idea of the varied roles she has had in her lifetime. Perhaps by listening to her views on being a wife, mother, sister, career woman, and so on, I can absorb more of what she really was and is, rather than the perception her halo has given me.

The narrowed perception precipitated by the halo effect is seldom rectified in evaluative isolation; we need the assistance of others in discussing that to which we are reacting and in attempting to correct it. Our interviews with patients are a source of information and give us an opportunity to test again and again the extent of our perceptions of patients. Regardless of whether a patient has a negative or positive halo effect, communicating thoughtfully and accurately with him during our interviews can broaden our perceptions of him and can abort the possible distorting influences of the halo effect upon our nursing care.

VARIABLE ERROR: VAGRANT OPINIONS

Variety in experiences, perceptions, thoughts, and feelings is the reason each of us is unique, and through it our lives are enriched and new insights are added to our perceptions. During these times we discover how differently several people can perceive the same object; this is called a variable error and is defined as the diversity of opinion held by several people about any single characteristic in another person. In nursing, variable errors occur often, but most frequently during morning report or other changes of shift, as indicated by the lively and frustrating discussions at these times.

The predicament these perceptions of a patient create is reminiscent of John Godfrey Saxe's parable *The Blind Men and the Elephant,* which is parodied in Figures 8 through 14 for purposes of illustration. The composite of the patient the nurses saw is presented in Figure 15.

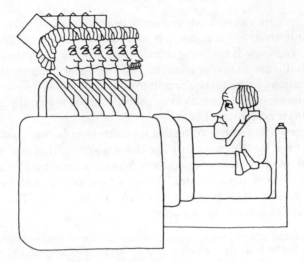

Fig. 8. It was six nurses of O-pin-i-an
to learning much inclined
Who went to see the Patient
(though most of them were blind)
that each by observation
might satisfy her mind.

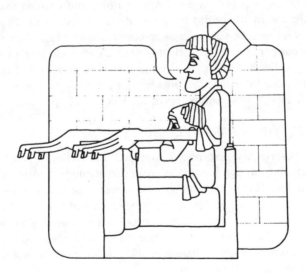

Fig. 9. The First approached the Patient and
happening to fall
against his broad and sturdy side,
at once began to bawl:
"God bless me! but this Patient is
very like a wall."

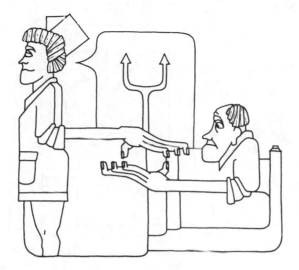

Fig. 10. The Second, feeling of the hand cried,
"Ho! What have we here. So very round
and smooth and sharp?
To me 'tis very clear, this wonder of a
Patient is very like a spear!"

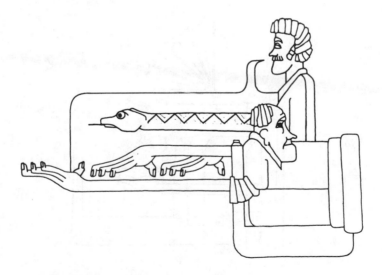

Fig. 11. The Third approached the Patient and
happening to take the squirming arm within
his hands
thus boldly up he spake:
"I see," quoth he, "the Patient is very like a snake!"

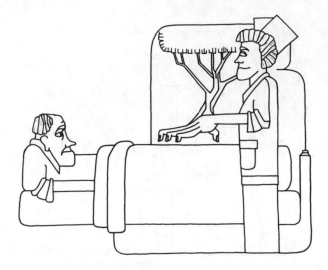

Fig. 12. The Fourth reached out an eager hand and
          felt about the knee:
          "What most this wondrous Patient is like
          is very plain, quoth she;
          "'Tis clear enough the Patient is very like a tree."

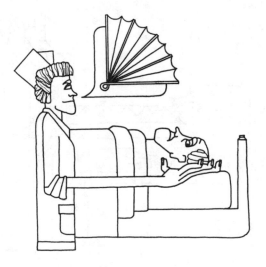

Fig. 13. The Fifth, who chanced to touch the ear,
          Said: "Even the blindest nurse
          can tell what this resembles most;
          Deny the fact who can, this marvel of a
          Patient is very like a fan!"

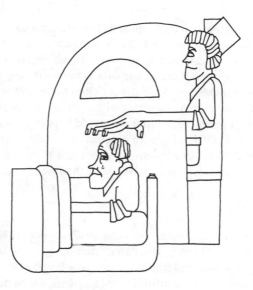

Fig. 14. The Sixth no sooner had begun
about the Patient to roam
Then coming to his moving head
that touched her fingerbone.
"I see," quoth she, "the Patient
Is very like a dome!"

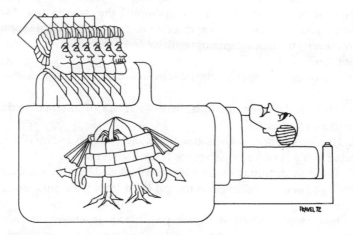

Fig. 15. What the nurses saw (composite view).

The different perceptions each nurse had of the same patient remind us of how different our perceptions are from those of our co-workers. Nevertheless, we manage to communicate with each other. In nursing, however, we must continue to have more exposure to and interactions with any patient who is the object of our variable errors. If the six blind nurses in the parody had exchanged places and each had contact with a different aspect of that patient, eventually through communication there would have been more accord about him. Our purpose in interacting with a patient is to gain a more complete picture of him. By sharing our impressions with those of our co-workers, we may yet discover that there is more to agree about than we may think.

SUMMARY

Attitudes are developed through a variety of experiences with other people. Together with what we have accumulated from our parents, they are the basis for our beliefs, thoughts, and feelings about people and events. Because we are generally unaware of how attitudes are acquired, we do not realize the need to question their validity. In nursing, however, the need for critically examining our attitudes is vital, because they affect our care of patients. Attitudes such as investment, acceptance, and objectivity can assist the patient by demonstrating our compassion for and commitment to his welfare. Attitudes such as condescension, forgetfulness, and lack of spontaneity obstruct such assistance. Common attitudinal perceptions, such as stereotyping, halo effects, and variable errors, exist because of our need to oversimplify the complexities of the world, its events, and its people. Becoming aware of these processes of simplification and correcting the misperceptions resulting from their use lend validity to our patient care.

Principles that emerge from this discussion of attitudes include the following:

1. Attitudes based on simplified beliefs and lack of information distort our perceptions of others.

2. Helping attitudes, such as investment, acceptance, and objectivity, are reflected in the conduct of each nurse toward each patient.

3. The individuality of each patient is threatened by attitudes that block his ability to understand, respond to, and learn from the events surrounding his care.

4. The degree to which we stereotype others is dependent on the extent to which our emotions are involved with the objects of our stereotyping.

5. Increasing the amount and quality of accurate information about any individual or group decreases the incidence of stereotypes, halo effects, and variable errors.

6. Communication behavior is altered to the degree that we evaluate the presence of stereotypes, halo effects, and variable errors in our relationships with patients.

NOTES

1. Triandis, Harry C. *Attitude and Attitude Change,* p. 5.
2. Combs, Arthur W. *Perceiving, Behaving, Becoming: A New Focus for Education,* p. 58.
3. McGregor, Frances C. *Social Science in Nursing,* pp. 46 and 70.
4. Kaiser Aluminum News. *Communications,* p. 39.
5. Gorden, Raymond L. *Interviewing: Strategy, Techniques and Tactics,* p. 221.
6. Triandis, op. cit. (note 1), pp. 102 and 103.
7. Bierce, Ambrose. *The Devil's Dictionary,* p. 49.
8. Triandis, op. cit. (note 1), p. 109.
9. Guilford, J. P. *Psychometric Methods,* p. 279.

BIBLIOGRAPHY

Bem, Daryl J. *Beliefs, Attitudes and Human Affairs.* Belmont, Calif.: Brooks Cole, 1970.
Bierce, Ambrose. *The Devil's Dictionary,* Reprint of 1906 ed. New York: Peter Pauper Press, 1958.
Combs, Arthur W. *Perceiving, Behaving, Becoming: A New Focus for Education.* Washington, D.C.: Association for Supervision and Curriculum Development, 1962.
Fishbein, Martin, ed. *Readings on Attitude Theory and Measurement.* New York: Wiley, 1967.
Freedman, Jonathan, Carlsmith, J. Merrill, and Sears, David. *Social Psychology.* Englewood Cliffs, N. J.: Prentice-Hall, 1970.
Gorden, Raymond. L. *Interviewing: Strategy, Techniques and Tactics.* Homewood, Ill.: Dorsey, 1969.
Guilford, J. P. *Psychometric Methods,* 2nd ed. New York: McGraw-Hill, 1954.
Halloran, James D. *Attitude Formation and Change.* Leicester, Great Britain: Leicester University Press, 1967.
Helmstradter, G. C. *Principles of Psychological Measurement.* New York: Appleton-Century-Crofts, 1964.
Kaiser Aluminum News. *Communications.* Oakland, Calif.: Kaiser Aluminum and Chemical Corporation, Vol. 23, No. 3, 1965.
McGregor, Frances C. *Social Science in Nursing.* New York: Wiley, 1960.
Triandis, Harry C. *Attitude and Attitude Change.* New York: Wiley, 1971.

8

Sociocultural Influences

IN OUR INTERACTIONS with others, each of us is the totality of conduct —
from all events, beliefs, and experiences that have preceded us. As cultural
messengers, we bring to others attitudes and conduct reminiscent of the past
but expressed in the idiom of the present. Through our activities and behavior
we influence and inform others about ourselves. In turn, we receive information
about others and are influenced by them. From this instinctive communicative
exchange, we provide ourselves with an encoding reservoir of thoughts, ideas,
and feelings from which to draw in the future.

Culture has purpose, which, as anthropologist Edward Hall believes, is to
generate itself among groups of people, so that their standards and ways of life
are supported and passed on as heritages [1]. These become so ingrained in
groups and individuals that they are not questioned or debated. Communication
is the medium by which our cultural heritage is maintained, conveyed, and translated as time passes. From this point of view, culture should invite, arouse, and
excite the curious individual to seek out and discover the ways in which his own
culture is expressed.

The hospital and the community provide us with settings in which to study
the ways people express their cultures. As contemporary nursing practice
extends into the community, there is less justification for nursing efforts that
are not grounded in an appreciation of the cultural elements communicated by
each member of the community and his family. Such efforts aid us to be aware
of our own cultural background, which influences our values and modes of
expression in our interactions with patients. The study of cultural elements such
as territoriality, privacy, time, waiting, and change can help us to become culturally aware of others as well as ourselves (Fig. 16).

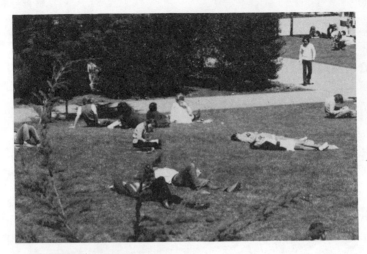

A. The space about us.

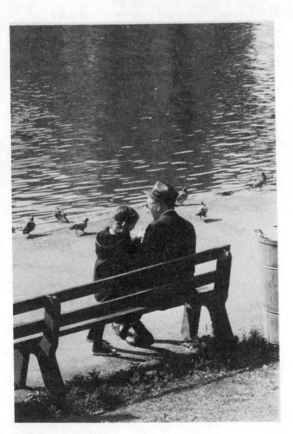

Fig. 16. Territoriality. The space about us can illustrate intimate distance, personal distance, social distance, public distance, or privacy. Architects and city planners consider such distances in constructing walking areas that can be used for communication.

B. Intimate distance.

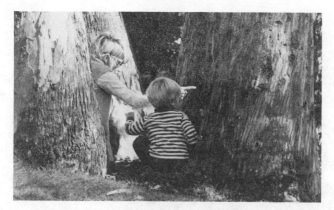

C. Personal distance.

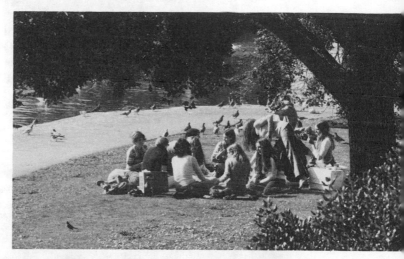

D. Social distance.

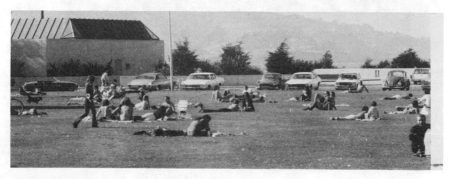

E. Public distance.

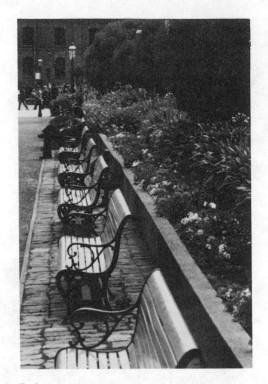

F. Privacy

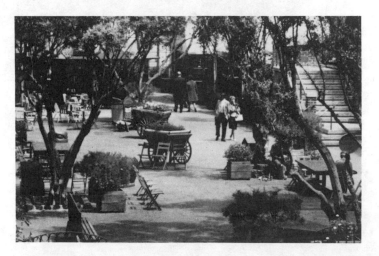

G. A setting constructed for use as a walking area.

TERRITORIALITY

Our behavior is guided by our culture. Nowhere is this more apparent than in our sense of personal space, that is, the distance at which we prefer to interact with others. With overcrowding of our population, our awareness of the use of space is heightened, and, as areas of space become more difficult to find and maintain, it is more difficult for us to preserve the autonomy of our personal space systems. The acquisition of land and property, the maintenance and protection of boundaries from intrusion, and the wealth and power derived from these acquisitions have historical antecedents in the life and behavior of us all.

Use of space and defense of territory were identified and described relative to animal behavior initially. Later, territoriality was applied to human behavior and defined as "that area of space about us which we possess and defend against intrusion from others" [2]. It is within the dimension of territory and space that we interact with others. Although the terms *territory* and *space* are often used interchangeably, a distinction should be made in terms of visibility and mobility [3]. Our personal space is mobile — it goes where we go — whereas territory, such as a house or a room, remains stationary. Territories can be separated and marked so that they are visible to others; a fence separates a sidewalk (public property) from a front yard (private property) in the same way a beach towel, beach bag, sandals, radio, and picnic basket mark off a territory on the beach (public property) we intend to use (as private property). Our personal space is invisible; our bodies are its center, and its dimension (that is, the place for interaction) is between our bodies and the walls of this invisible barrier.

When these boundaries are threatened by intrusion, our communication alters in direct response to it. Whatever our cultural orientation to both space and territory, the same message conveyed from varying distances assumes different meanings and underlying motives. The closer or more imminent the threat, the stronger the need to overtly display defensive communication behavior. We may not be aware of our defensive attitude within the dimension of personal space, but our contact with other people, as Hall points out, demonstrates its presence and the variety of ways space is organized in each culture [4]. The behavior communicated to people of various cultural persuasions through our use of space in nursing practice requires exploration.

THE DISTANCES WE KEEP

Since our communication alters in proportion to the distance we keep from others, a brief description of the four types of distances, as delineated by Hall [5], that affect communication is necessary. These areas for interaction are determined by the nature of the relationship, what we are doing at the time, and the perceptions and feelings related to the relationship and to the task at hand.

Intimate distance is characterized by two phases, close and far, which extend from zero to eighteen inches. The sensation experienced by most of us at this distance is overwhelming, and the presence of the other person is unmistakable. In the close phase (zero to six inches), body contact is inevitable and expected. Sensory detection is heightened and distorted because of the increased input of stimuli, such as body heat and smell. Musculature is active and the two people seek physical contact with each other. Visual detail is sharpened, and such closeness pulls the eyes into a cross-eyed position, which is unique to this distance. Vocalizations that do occur are involuntary and play a minor role at this point.

As the distance of intimacy extends to its far phase of six to eighteen inches, vocalization becomes low and is more frequent. Although musculature is still active and anticipatory, the participants are not in close approximation, though their hands are in easy reach of each other. Visual focus is easier, though the objects in range, such as the head, and aspects of the face, seem distorted and larger than they really are. Body heat and smell are still perceptible, even though they are directed away from the other person.

Personal distance resembles an invisible shield that protects us from physical contact with other people. This protective area of one and one-half to four feet includes a close phase of one and one-half to two and one-half feet and a far phase of two and one-half to four feet. In the close phase, close physical contact is possible by holding or grasping the other person, but in the far phase, only touching is possible. Here, our physical domination is severely curtailed, visual perception involves less distortion, and facial details, as one example, are clearer. There is a three-dimensional quality to the people we see. Our stance and vocal tone clearly establish the type of personal relationship and the meaning it may have for us and for others. As personal distance is extended to four feet, we shift our gaze over the face rather than focus on a part of the face, such as an eye or the mouth. Voice levels at this distance are moderate, and body heat and smell are not as perceptible.

Social distance, four to twelve feet, includes a close phase of four to seven feet and a far phase of seven to twelve feet. It denotes a limit to the degree of physical domination exerted by one person over another. At this distance, we are screened and protected from others without having to resort to rudeness. At the same time, it permits us the opportunity to conduct business without the intensity of closer spatial distances. There are few differences between the close and far phases of social distance. Our visual perception is clearer and includes more, although fine detail, such as facial imperfections, is lost. Eye contact becomes important at this distance, and since we visually incorporate the entire face of the other person, we need not shift our gaze back and forth from eye to mouth to maintain contact with them. The whole figure of the person whom we are facing is perceived, though body heat and odor are not. Vocalization becomes louder and can be overheard by others. Interactions at this distance generally are more formal, though there is more involvement between people within the closer phase.

Beyond the twelve-foot perimeter of social distance is an area considered vacant of personal involvement with others. This is called *public distance* and ranges from twelve to twenty-five feet in the close phase, and from twenty-five feet to infinity in the far phase. Loud vocalization and careful pronunciation are required when speaking. In doing so, subtlety of meaning is lost, and the facial expressions used to convey it are not readily perceptible. All movement and expressiveness, therefore, must be exaggerated or amplified. Details, such as the color of the eyes, so apparent in previous distances, are less noticeable at this distance. Although the faces of other people can be seen in the close phase of public distance, their distinctiveness as humans steadily decreases as public distances increase.

PRIVACY: OUR PERSONAL IMPERATIVE

As the world becomes more crowded, more impersonal, and filled with more sensory stimuli than we have ever known, the desire for privacy becomes less whimsical and more imperative. The protection of this spatial prerogative involves more ritualistic activity in the acquisition and use of personal space. Because of our need to voluntarily withdraw physically or psychologically from others, seeking privacy is a valuable autonomous act. Indeed, this exercise of autonomy, that is, the development and preservation of our individuality, is a basic function of privacy.

Every time we withdraw from others we provide ourselves the opportunity to engage in other activities conducted in privacy, namely, emotional release and self-evaluation. Such moments afford us the opportunity not only to siphon off pent-up feelings due to the stresses and pressures of daily living, but also to evaluate the extent and validity of the feelings being released. When this is difficult or impossible, privacy takes the form of limited or protected communication, in which our feelings and confidences can be shared with selected people who, by the nature of their role or function, are bound not to share our disclosures with others [6].

There are two ways in which privacy and its associated activities can be initiated. Spatially, the easiest and most visible way is by the physical manipulation of objects in our environment. Closing the door of our room, going for a drive, not answering the telephone, or leaving a crowded room clearly demonstrates our wish to be alone. Through our actions we insure the physical protection necessary to maintain our privacy in the space we have arranged for ourselves. Providing we are among others of our own culture, our wish for privacy usually is respected. Such may not be the case among people whose cultural orientation to privacy differs markedly.

Escapes into privacy are necessary at some time for us all, not only for release and evaluation of our feelings, but also for the solace of solitude. From this state of privacy, the genesis of any creative force emerges and fills us with a feeling that theologian Paul Tillich describes as the joy of being alone [7].

Despite our attempts to achieve privacy through physical withdrawal and manipulation of our environment, we may not be successful. The alternative is our personal space bubble, which can be used even in the presence of others. This intrapsychic maneuver (that is, the activation of behavioral forces within the self) is exquisitely communicated through our nonverbal behavior. Our faces become vacant of expression, we stare without seeing, our thoughts and feelings encapsulated in bodies propelled in movement or hunched while sitting all communicate a wish to be left alone — protected by self-induced anonymity in order to secure a measure of privacy for ourselves.

NURSES, PATIENTS, AND THE DISTANCES BETWEEN

Our starting point is to translate the sociocultural elements of territoriality and privacy to nursing and to observe their use both in the hospital and in the community. The types of distances previously mentioned will serve as the context of this discussion.

Intimate Distance: Close as a Whisper

We interact at intimate distances with patients in the hospital in both planned and unplanned physical contact. Both approaches are appropriate in our professional role. The nestling of a newborn infant in our arms is instinctive (in moments of affection) and necessary (relative to feeding). Warmth from our bodies and physical contact with us are necessary stimuli for the newborn.

Another nursing measure often used in hospitals is personal restraint, in which our bodies are used to block a patient's actions, particularly if they may be destructive or injurious to him. Physically securing a child by holding him when he is given an intramuscular injection is one example. The physical restraint used to guide body movements during convulsive seizures, the restraint used during acute distress in patients with emotional problems, and the calming restraint used with patients thrashing about in bed as a result of high fever are other examples of how we implement the space of intimate distance in our nursing practice.

Intimate distance is also used in nursing activities that deal with the intimacy of body functions. The nursing of unconscious patients and those who are conscious but confined to bed involves the management of their excretory processes.

Emergencies may require the intimate distance between ourselves and our patients to be closed dramatically, such as during mouth-to-mouth resuscitation or cardiac arrest.

Physical support also involves intimate distance. Patients requiring the physical security of our arms in helping them to get up in bed or into a chair illustrate this point. Positioning unconscious or severely injured conscious patients also involves a great deal of body contact.

Often the way we verbally communicate with our patients at these times reflects an instinctive awareness of the need to adjust the tone of our voice to the distance we are using. Keeping auditory contact with an unconscious patient, for example, requires a soft yet clear voice, because although he may suffer a variety of sensory impairments, his hearing may still be intact. A loud voice may overwhelm him and inhibit his ability to sort the verbal input he receives. Decreasing the volume of our voices, speaking distinctly, and using words and statements that are simple and easily understood have a reassuring and calming effect on patients who may interpret loudness, urgency, rapidity, and complexity of speech with a worsening of their illness.

While a patient is receiving nursing care he may be observing how we are utilizing this distance. His perception of us is based largely upon what he learns of us visually. Since illness alters the sensory mechanisms of patients, the sensory perceptions they receive, while seemingly uneventful to us, are frequently heightened or distorted.

Visiting people in their homes adds insight into the ways distances are used and communicated to us. We are received as guests, visiting a territory as new to us as the hospital must be to our patients. Here, in the comfort and security of their homes, the individuals and families are freer in the communication they share with us. Young children, after their inspection of us from behind their mothers, usually become eager for attention and often wish to come into closer physical contact with us. Depending on the trust established in our relationship with them, older people often express their affection through the closeness of intimate distance. By offering support through a comforting embrace, we can express what words cannot.

As a helping relationship develops, we can see and understand how distance is used by the people and families we visit. The reduction of distance alone indicates an interpersonal closeness that may not have been present previously. Since we are guests in someone else's territory, the move to reduce spatial distance is his prerogative. Sometimes this is done innocuously, as when we are shown family picture albums or scrapbooks filled with mementos of an earlier more active life. Contact achieved through these means is not only less threatening to both parties, but the items used also provide a neutral ground in which to test how one will be received at this close distance.

Intimate distance is not maintained throughout home visits; it is attained occasionally and indicates an emotional component operating either within the relationship, or outside it but being discharged within the visit. Our instinctive response to prolonged use of intimate distance is to move away when we begin to feel threatened or uncomfortable. Our feelings and attitudes about our own intimate distance must be explored, especially if such discomfort is not demonstrated in the person we are visiting. Feelings of discomfort are not uncommon when we visit sightless people who rely on physical contact, or deaf people to whom it is also important.

Relationship to Privacy. A natural instinct for us all is to maintain and protect the space immediately surrounding us, which has been identified as intimate distance, a space we share with our families and other selected people. Each time we make such a decision, we exercise personal autonomy in deciding who is and who is not to be admitted into this intimate proximity. We thereby reinforce our self-concept in deciding how we use the space that encircles us.

The hospital, however, drastically curtails a patient's autonomy with respect to his body and his personal space. He is verbally prodded with personal questions asked by strangers who, in addition, physically and visually invade his body during examination. These acts of invasion are permitted because they reflect the special status conferred upon doctors and nurses within their professional roles, which permits the rules of privacy to be waived. Such emphasis on prestige, authority, or technical skills is necessary "in order to protect the self from the shame which ordinarily accompanies a revelation of the body to a stranger" [8]. This is the mechanism that permits us access to the intimate space bubble of our patients and allows them to tolerate our close proximity.

We too are protected from the cultural offense of such intimate access to patients. In a sense, we mask ourselves in the garb of a professional stranger, taking care not to communicate behaviors that are not a part of that role or a part of our cultural orientation to privacy.

Our major task in reinforcing our patients' right to privacy is to afford them every opportunity possible in which to exercise autonomy in their intimate space. This includes not only participation in decision-making, but also physical manipulation of their personal possessions to reinforce the areas over which they have control. With their personal identity threatened, the anonymity of hospital life, the absence of their possessions, the loss of continuity with familiar territory, and their body under professional scrutiny and under assault by illness, both the need for security and for privacy are expressed in terms of the familiar, through identification and manipulation of what is their own — their possessions and the guaranteed use of the space to which they have been assigned.

By anticipating this need, we can assist them in having their personal belongings within easy reach — approximately eighteen inches. Physiologically this lessens the physical exertion required by patients with cardiac problems, for example. Psychologically, by meeting the expectations for space and privacy, it lessens the psychic energies patients have to exert in the preservation of their autonomy.

Marking off territory that defines their space bubble, such as in intimate distance, is one way of insuring it. The seemingly inconsequential requests or the demands our patients make regarding the closeness of their personal belongings, therefore, should not go unheeded. Privacy, already limited by shortages of space in a hospital, is a luxury for most patients. Whenever possible, privacy, especially concerning a patient's body and the immediate space around it, should be preserved and respected by each of us.

Personal Distance: A Place of Confidences

In the hospital, we are more at ease using personal distance in our contacts with patients, because we can move nearer to or away from the patient without expressing acute discomfort. Various nursing tasks affirm this flexibility; they use some physical contact with patients but also allow us to interact without physical contact if necessary. They may include giving injections and other medications, sitting with or bathing a patient, or checking intravenous feedings.

Personal distance is most conducive to refining our observations of patients since we are apt to see more of their features without necessarily resorting to touch. We also become less threatening and overwhelming to them because we are less distorted.

The flexibility possible within personal distance provides for the interpersonal closeness necessary to the development of helping relationships. Communication within this distance can alternate between purposeful sharing of thoughts and feelings, characteristic of the close phase, and less involved, conversational banter, which is characteristic of the far phase. This distance facilitates more sharing, because our appearance and actions are less imposing and intense than at intimate distance.

Again, home visits provide a natural setting for the use of personal distance. Seating arrangements usually are within this distance, thereby making the subjects under discussion more personal and reciprocal. Shaking hands is often a preliminary ritual that communicates how both participants react to each other within this distance. If the chairs are not usually in close proximity, often the family sees that they are rearranged for the visit. Where we are seated in relation to the usual seating placement of the person we are visiting communicates a great deal in terms of the use of personal space at this distance. For example:

> Mrs. F., a slight 83-year-old black woman, was visited every three weeks by a young nursing student of Filipino origin. Every visit was begun with directions concerning the seating arrangements. The student was guided to a small straight-back chair approximately three feet opposite a

large rocking chair, where the elderly lady sat during the visits. Midway between the chairs and off to one side was a 30-year-old plant, which Mrs. F. had named Mary. After the visit, the student remarked in her conference: "I keep getting the feeling there are three of us visiting together: Mrs. F., me, and Mary. I wonder if Mrs. F. talked with her children in this way."

Personal distance is often utilized in the seating arrangements in out-patient clinics and other visiting rooms, but crowding in these areas may promote non-contact and noninvolvement. Taking walks with the elderly we visit and observing children of the families we visit at play in their yards or at nursery schools give us an overview to the uses of personal distance by a variety of cultures and to the rules that govern spatial conduct during these times.

Relationship to Privacy. One of the functions of privacy that is best served within personal distance is limited and protected communication. Our status as professionals has already been established or initiated in actions involving intimate distance. As we retreat to the less overwhelming noncontact distance, we offer our patients more opportunity to share with us their concerns and problems, but the personal distance sphere in a hospital or a home does not necessarily guarantee privacy. Few places in a hospital, for example, lend themselves to privacy, especially if a patient is in a ward of four or more beds. In the home, family demands often interrupt the best intentioned efforts to initiate the sharing of confidential matters. Regardless of the setting, and because of the responsibility to insure our patients' privacy, we are "subject to definite obligations regarding both the manner in which secret knowledge is to be obtained and, most importantly, the way in which it is treated once it has been obtained" [9].

At this distance we are better able to see any nonverbal behaviors that may signal a psychological tuning out of the topic under discussion or of conversation in general. These psychological barriers raised in search of privacy even in the presence of others is readily observable in many health settings; the patient is huddled in the middle of his invisible sphere, reconnoitering his thoughts and problems. During these moments, interruptions may seem intrusive. The proximity we have maintained can serve us well if we use it to observe whether the barriers continue to be raised against interpersonal intrusions, thereby indicating the degree of receptivity if we wish to communicate.

Efforts to facilitate a helping relationship commonly are made within this distance in the form of interpersonal communication. Our physical proximity alone indicates our availability and readiness to assist the patient in some helpful or productive way. The thoughts and inquiries we may pursue indicate our psychological presence and investment as well.

Privacy is a commodity in a hospital and a scarce one at that. It is obtained for a price — the cost of a private room. Since most rooms in a hospital are not private, scarcity creates demand. Certain criteria determine the priorities for its occupants. Serious, terminal, and contagious illness are compelling physiological reasons for the use of private rooms, but being able to afford them often takes priority.

The ability to purchase privacy reflects the position or status of the purchaser in our society. The higher his status, the more control he has over the amount and kind of privacy he has. Unfortunately, people from cultural minority groups, the indigent and the uneducated who may or may not live in crowded ghettos, do not have the status or the money to obtain the privacy they may wish for themselves.

Despite the difficulty in achieving total privacy in a hospital, there are things that we can do to insure the privacy of our patients' territorial boundaries. Placing screens around a bed or drawing the curtains around it insures visual privacy and indicates clearly to other patients and staff in the room that whatever is to take place within the prescribed boundary is a private matter, regardless of whether it involves a nursing procedure or an interview.

At times, a television, radio, and voices of people in the room provide a cover of sound that interferes with the ability to hear what is being discussed. Lowering our voices or closing the distance between ourselves and the patient indicates our recognition of a patient's right to share his thoughts with privacy. If the patient is ambulatory, moving to a more private area may be indicated.

The home is a setting more natural and conducive to the exercise of autonomy; it represents a person's ability to exert control of his privacy. How each person conducts himself within his sphere of personal distance communicates his ability to influence and control his environment. This is a strong need in all of us and one difficult to relinquish, because it would mean the decline or cessation of one's independence in action and in decision-making. Such was the case of the 83-year-old woman in the following example:

> During her home visits with a nursing student, Mrs. F. always sat in her big rocker, which commanded the room from its vantage point near the window. The lady was in failing health and had to rest in bed a great deal. When the nursing student arrived, Mrs. F. told her to sit in her rocker, which was the first time she had done this. After a while, Mrs. F. said to the student, "You've never seen me in this position before, have you?" The student realized that the woman was not only talking about her failing health but also referring to the loss of her autonomy, which she had always communicated by sitting in "her" chair and directing others to their chairs and the use of space within her apartment. Mrs. F's comments acknowledged a change of roles between them. She had become more dependent upon the student as a helping person who was able and decisive.

As trust develops in a helping relationship, the boundaries of privacy in a home may be lifted and extended over a period of time. For example, additional rooms may be made accessible to us. Visits may be held in the kitchen, where personal distance is maintained by sitting at the kitchen table. The distance created by the table still permits sharing (even food), yet does not inhibit communication. Access to other rooms may be additional demonstrations of trust, but this occurs gradually. The concepts of personal property and privacy are strong cultural derivatives, which must be respected, regardless of the frustration.

> Mrs. J. was a woman of Portuguese background, whose excessive weight limited her movements. Each time the nursing student paid a call, Mrs. J. was sitting in the same chair, facing the television, which was always on, even during the visit. The student was directed to either a chair or a hassock a few feet to the left of Mrs. J., since a TV tray was at her right. Despite the range of topics discussed and the student's subtle hints to see the house, Mrs. J. made no move to show it to her. If Mrs. J. wanted something to drink, she would ask her daughter, who was in the kitchen most of the time, to bring it, despite the student's willingness to get it. Only after a year had gone by and the student was making her final visits did Mrs. J. allow her to help the daughter prepare some tea in the kitchen.

The trust a person extends to us may be demonstrated through the distance we maintain as well as through the promises we make and keep and the confidences we guard and hold. Movement from one distance sphere to another may be first communicated nonverbally. Trust can also be withdrawn, as in the following example:

> Mrs. Z. and a nursing student began their visits and their relationship by sitting opposite each other at a distance of eight or nine feet. As their relationship developed, Mrs. Z. began to seat herself nearer the student. At first she moved her chair closer, but later she sat on the sofa with the student. Often their visits took place in the kitchen, where the closer proximity was continued. During the last two visits of the year, the student observed that Mrs. Z. had returned to the chair she sat in at the beginning of the year. Although the visits continued to be friendly and warm, they were, nevertheless, conducted from this distance.

Trust, autonomy, observation of nonverbal behavior, and limited and protected communication, whatever the locale, are the aspects of privacy most likely to be achieved within personal distance in helping relationships. Use of that space must be carefully observed and guided if we are to include it, with its cultural variations, in our nursing practice.

Social Distance: Out of Reach

Activity is the dominant theme of social distance in hospital life; it is exemplified by movement back and forth between nurses and patients. We can see the "limit of domination" unfolding in several aspects of hospital life where interactions occur with groups of people or staff. Accompanying an intern or resident on rounds, passing out medication to large numbers of patients in a ward, chatting in a doorway, and saying hello or waving to patients in the solarium represent instances in which social distance is used. The purpose of social distance is to provide expediency in dealing with several patients at one time. It lends an aura of presence without the necessity of physical contact. Seeing and hearing, *not* touching, are the primary forms of communication during encounters with patients. With the large number of patients in hospital wards, and our increasing responsibility for their care, social distance is important because it offers a means of completing our work without involving ourselves personally and intensively with every patient. Limited involvement describes our interactions with patients within this sphere, and it is protective for both ourselves and our patients, because it reduces the amount of sensory bombardment.

A nursing station is a pocket of space that also represents the limit of domination and protects our territorial boundary from intrusion of patients. They may approach it and lean on it, but they are not permitted into it. This is understood, yet the visual and vocal interaction here remains generally pleasant and informal.

Group situations in the hospital and community created for a specific purpose also involve social distance. In the circle formed in group therapy, social distance is the space *between* group members sitting opposite each other; members sitting *next* to each other are closer. Aside from encounter groups using touch extensively, social distance in other gatherings is activated through vocal and visual modes of expression. Although touch may play a part in these situations, it is not a primary source of contact. Members of nontherapy groups for political activity, senior citizens, health teaching, and vocational rehabilitation, for example, function within this sphere. Families as a group also use social distance, but the purpose and duration fluctuate.

Relationship to Privacy. The limit of domination implied by social distance poses a danger to the privacy we wish to establish for ourselves and our patients. Social distance, with its limited involvement between people, sets the stage for a limited presentation of ourselves. We show selected aspects of our personality, attitudes, and feelings to others whose relationship to us is also restricted and selective. In a work-oriented setting, this may be necessary in order that we do not become distracted with the personal details of our co-workers' lives. To an extent this is protective, because indiscriminate and personal revelations about ourselves may be ego-stripping and may alienate us from others. For every behavior we share with others in social and in public distance, there are other behaviors that remain the exclusive domain of more intimate spatial distances. Such balance has a stabilizing effect on our personalities.

This limit of personal and physical domination is appropriate as long as it does not inflict anonymity, that penalty of privacy which may become a threat to our ego-identity. Anonymity, or the absence of a specific identity, is characterized by freedom from public expectation, that is, freedom from behaviors or actions that ordinarily are supervised or open to the comments and criticism of others. If anonymity is intense and perpetuated over a prolonged period, dehumanization is likely.

Patients are subjected daily to threats and feelings of anonymity. Although they had some control over the extent of it outside the hospital, the choice is not as apparent *in* an institutional setting. As long as autonomy can be exerted in other aspects of life, the anonymity of walking on a crowded sidewalk or standing in line, and the indignity of having to prove or establish our identity in trying to cash a check, can be tolerated with civility.

Initiated to the invasion of privacy through the personal questions asked in the admitting department and continued by members of the staff, patients soon become uncomfortably accustomed to being identified by their hospital number, room number, or type of disease. One unfortunate habit we have is assigning them nonhuman or anonymous nicknames, as reflected in these comments: "She's a doll"; "He's growling like a bear this morning"; "She looks like a stick"; "Compared to the others, he's a bull in a china shop", or "Room 114, Bed A."

When we use these terms among ourselves, we can only speculate the effect of our attitudes and feelings on patients. We are often repaid in kind when they fail to remember our names, functions, and titles. The number of staff members our patients encounter daily and the limited involvement allowed by the social distance used by them also reinforce feelings of anonymity.

The community perhaps is even more pervasive in this respect. Nowhere is this more evident than in the downtown hotel lobbies housing our aged. In many of these lobbies, for example, chairs are grouped in a semicircle within the social distance limits, but not so far apart that a conversation could not be maintained. The patrons, however, do not utilize the space for interaction, except if necessary or expedient. All the more poignant is the fact that often the same people occupy the same spatial territory day after day, and yet their only interaction may be visual intake, barely acknowledged by other nonverbal behavior. This is pathetically similar to mental patients of large state institutions, who are often known by the places they keep rather than the people they are. These individuals are not benefiting from even the limited involvement possible in this captive socialization area. They require interpersonal involvement activated by closer spatial proximity.

Where spatial territories are unattractive (in decor), unvarying (in routine), unchanging (in attitude), uncommunicative (in behavior), and unremitting (in monotony), new space will be claimed, however temporary. To the elderly, whose possessions and territorial boundaries decrease over the years, the instinct to defend whatever territory they acquire becomes fiercely accentuated. For example, one particular chair in a lobby becomes an instinctual issue to be defended and guarded from newcomers.

The behavior of territorial defense can be directed into channels that will encourage social involvement within this spatial distance, as in the following interaction:

> Mrs. O. had been institutionalized for twenty years. Her English was very limited, though she could understand more than she admitted. Her pattern of behavior seldom deviated from the privately enforced routine she had established. Aside from her meals, she seldom ventured beyond her bedroom area and was often forgotten by other patients and staff. She would either walk the length of the sleeping dormitory or occupy herself with small tasks in the vicinity of her own bed. Although she smiled or nodded to others from a distance, she became increasingly tense and anxious if anyone new came near her or her bed. If they came within six feet of it, she began talking loudly in her native language and shook her fist at the intruder. She became calmer when they retreated.
>
> A nursing student who had observed this behavior decided to visit Mrs. O. on a regular basis and began her visits by sitting three beds away from Mrs. O. The student carefully observed the distance between Mrs. O. and herself and proceeded slowly to reduce it. By the end of six weeks, the student was able to place her chair at the foot of the bed next to Mrs. O. without receiving any verbal reaction. Occasionally Mrs. O. would invite the student to sit on her bed in order to show her something. By the end of the tenth week, the two of them walked to the lounge for their visit, but a distance of four to five feet was still being maintained.

In this example, the relationship began at the far phase of social distance and was eventually reduced to the close phase. Later in the relationship, the distance between them was reduced even more, but these actions were initiated by the patient, who apparently felt comfortable and trusted the student sufficiently to do so. The socialization of Mrs. O. continued to be slow, but it was basic to the development of the relationship.

Behaviors in defense of our territory and privacy often become exaggerated as the reason for the protection becomes obscured. The same behaviors are used whenever the security provided by anonymity is threatened.

> Miss C., aged 71, has lived alone since the death of her mother five years ago. She joined the nearby senior center and has been able to socialize, but she does not linger with people long enough to do more than exchange amenities. She never invites people into her home and avoids those who suggest it. On several occasions when she conversed with a nursing student, she was able to sit quietly next to the student for ten to fifteen minutes, or as long as the conversation dealt with other people or events. Whenever the discussion began to focus on herself, her home, or her personal

opinions, she promptly got up and extended the distance between them by about ten feet. She remained here until she calmed down and then returned to the chair next to the student.

This lady used social distance as a means of relieving her anxiety and protecting her privacy (that is, anonymity).

Though anonymity is a degree of privacy we all use and protect, it is not desirable if it severely impairs the ability to form and maintain the socialization skills fundamental to all interpersonal relationships. Social distance provides the sphere for this socialization, and success within it often is the basis upon which closer relationships are formed. Remaining uninvolved is often a prologue to diminishing social interaction. People then become frozen in a spatial prison that has already constricted their involvement. Clearly, these people, whether in a hospital or the community, need to be reached in the space they occupy and moved into a less socially constricting area. Our efforts to establish helping relationships with these people are a means to that end.

Public Distance and the Distant Public

Distance separates, and as it does so, physical contact and social exchange become more remote and more difficult to achieve. What was a finely etched detail in close proximity becomes a broad impressionistic brushstroke as the distance increases, merely suggesting detail in place of detail. This is public distance, a distance vacant of personal, physical, and social proximity.

As distance separates us more and more from others, it creates illusions — a "cluster of notions" [10] perceived and experienced by us as reality. Opinions and attitudes derived from such notions are misleading because they do not represent an accurate picture of the real world.

The community is within the domain of public distance. Over the years, we too have formed a "cluster of notions" about the community and use the term *as if* it represented one person instead of many people. This is infinitely easier because, as mentioned previously, people within public distance begin to lose their individual features and proportions. Personal and family needs, hopes, and concerns, therefore, become blurred and are replaced by countless statistics and overused generalizations that support an overall picture of the community.

Each community is made up of smaller communities representing a common cultural background and socioeconomic level. Their interests and needs are diverse and are coined in the communication of that culture. Nursing also represents a subculture. It has a setting (traditionally the hospital), a language, customs, and status. Brought together in the public distance called the community, we are apt to find that we, as nurses, are more distant than we care to be, because in coming to the community, we discover that we do not know the cultural territory or the language, its customs, or its people. At the same time, we discover that the people do not know about our nursing culture and the way we express it. The result is a cultural isolationism, which increases physical and social distance through the misperception of intent, communication, and life style of other cultures. When each of us views our nursing practice in terms of what *we* feel is needed, and this in turn is based upon our own cultural beliefs and background, we are *increasing* rather than decreasing the psychological distances with respect to nursing practice.

Relationship to Privacy. The result of more distance between ourselves, as professional nurses, and individuals and families of the community we hope to help is a dichotomy, which Hoggart calls the world of "them" [11]. Because privacy is diminishing and feelings of alienation and anonymity are increasing, subgroups and subcultures view each other with suspicion. The community becomes a strange place — unrewarding and unhelpful. A feeling of aloneness is experienced, similar to the feelings expressed in the following lines:

> Distance
> is where we were
> but empty of us and ahead of
> me lying out in the rushes . . . .
> When I stop I am alone [12].*

This strange world of community has all the chips stacked on its side. Hoggart describes the world of "them" as:

> . . . a world of bosses, whether those bosses are private individuals or public officials . . . "them" includes policemen . . . [*social workers, landlords, doctors, nurses*] . . . whom working classes meet . . . to the very poor [*or to people and families in need*] especially, they compose a shadowy but numerous and powerful group affecting their lives at almost every point . . . "they are the people at the top" . . . who . . . "get yer in the end" . . . "aren't really to be trusted", "are all in a clique together", "treat y' like muck" [13].

Strange as these attitudes are, they exist *here* in our community — they exist *now* in our community and they *will continue* to exist as long as the cultural disparity between ourselves as nurses and the people whose care is our responsibility is reinforced. When we place ourselves in such a position through our limited understanding of what reality is in a community, we stand accused of being one of "them." The ideal proximity would be one in which we stood face to face with those families and individuals to transact the business of health and

---

*From "Words from a Totem Animal," in *The Carrier of Ladders* by W. S. Merwin. Copyright © 1967, 1970 by W. S. Merwin. Reprinted by permission of Atheneum Publishers.

health care from points of matched perceptions and knowledge of each others' cultural reality. The lives in our community need not remain hidden from or anonymous to us, just as our function as sincere and concerned nurses need not be obscured, even at this distance.

TIME AND WAITING

Space has already been identified as the *place* used either privately or publicly for interaction between ourselves and others. The events that take place in these locations and the behavior that results therein are coordinated by another culturally determined concept — time. Within the dimensions of space, time is a temporal boundary, which gives our social behavior sequential order and relates this order to the event taking place. The assumptions and definitions of time are determined by our culture and are reflected in our actions with others. Our views concerning punctuality, the use or waste of time, as well as the lack and value of it, demonstrate the extent to which it influences us, as one element of culture.

The concept of time has its cultural counterpart — waiting. This is an act of temporal expectation; waiting acts as a staying element in which some behavior, person, or event is anticipated within the boundary of time. Given the symbols of time (e.g., clocks, newspapers, calendars, light, and darkness), waiting becomes an act of measuring the duration, sequence, and passage of time, thereby determining its meaning to us. Nursing practice is within this temporal dimension; therefore, the functions of time and waiting need to be examined carefully for the implications they hold for nursing.

TIME AND TIME INTERVALS: USES AND MEANING FOR PATIENTS

Time as Social Meaning

During our interactions with patients, time acquires a social meaning, which is accumulated from memories and cultural interpretations of past uses of time. In turn, these activate and determine our actions and behavior with other people.

Within a hospital, for instance, time takes on more meaning because of the location. The time during which a patient is ill reactivates previous memories and behavior connected with illness. Although we are culturally oriented to looking forward in time, it is also a dimension of the past, because what we experience and see around us has already occurred.

It is worth remembering that actually we never see or experience anything *but* the past. The sounds you are hearing now come from a thousandth of a second back in time for every foot they have to travel to reach your ears.

What is true of sound is also true of light, though on a scale almost exactly a million times shorter. When we look out into space we can see events that occurred centuries or even millions of years ago [14].

Depending on our moods, especially in a hospital, these experiences of sight and sound may differ; time may seem to rush by or to linger too long. The feelings and attitudes recalled from the past in relation to illness are reenacted in the present hospital experience.

These feelings and attitudes may involve dependency needs, relationships with figures of authority, loss of status, and fear of death among patients. Although the reactivated feelings vary, they usually are not static. When a patient is placed within the confined space of a hospital, the temporal dimension telescopes specific factors of his past and assigns them social meaning, which is then expressed through the various modes and media of communication.

Time as a Fixed Resource

The extent to which time acquires social meaning in the hospital gives us insight into its use as a fixed resource. As such we are acknowledging that as a dimension of the past, time and its segments (minutes, hours, days, and so forth) cannot be restored once they have been used. Culturally, we place great emphasis on the uses of time. Its value creates scarcity, and scarcity increases its value, which clichés such as "time is money" bear out. The more tasks we have to perform within a given time segment, the more precious time becomes. The rapidity or slowness with which it passes is greatly influenced by the number of tasks involved in a time segment.

Time as a fixed resource is an observable element of a temporal dimension. Segmenting time into rigid schedules programmed as patient care (sometimes irreverently called nursing care plans) is one outstanding example. Certain times or schedules are set for bathing patients, for administering medications, for distributing meals, and for allowing sleep. Should any one of these routines or schedules be altered or deviated from, we discover through the communication from our co-workers that the schedule was too "heavy" and there was too much to be done in the time allotted, which is then used as a rationalization, justifying why something was not done for a patient.

As we set our time priorities relative to patients and tasks, we communicate them to our patients. They soon learn, for example, to make their requests known while we are with them. In addition, patients often feel they must apologize for having taken up our time because they know that we are busy, an attitude that often extends into family visits in the community. Our priorities of time often give patients the impression that they (as people) are not as high on the list as the tasks related to their illness.

Another perception of time as a valuable fixed resource is that the more time spent with one patient, the sicker he must be and the less there is to give to other patients. Realistically, sicker patients do require more of our time, and this priority does reinforce the impression that the sicker he is, the more likely he will get to see the nurse. Patients who may not be as sick as others may need more of our time than they receive, but sensing the different value placed upon it in the hospital, they hesitate to intrude upon it. This attitude may have defeated the goals for progressive patient care introduced several years ago.

Time as a Temporal Setting

Time also serves as a temporal setting for events in our lives; each event in which we participate assumes a meaning based on a particular setting. For example, the *Victorian era* is the term used for the temporal setting of the mid-nineteenth century. Against this backdrop, customs, manners, and morals assumed a meaning characteristic of the period; strict social and moral codes, male supremacy, and class consciousness are a few.

To judge an interaction or event with accuracy or perspective, we must consider the temporal setting of the people involved. Consequently, it would be unfair of us to dismiss the indignation of an elderly person who, for example, strongly disapproves of young couples living together without benefit of a legal marriage. By dismissing the attitude as unreasonable or not "with the times," we are judging him from our own temporal setting of the twentieth century, and forgetting that all his behaviors, attitudes, and feelings have been tempered by another social era. Subsequently, his values should be considered against the backdrop of his temporal setting.

The informal use of language in our country, even among relative strangers, is not fully appreciated by people who were brought up in another time and place. Regardless of the reason for it, such as language difficulties, attitudes, or lack of respect for others, the fundamental problem is a difference in temporal settings. We take our attitudes and customs for granted because they are reinforced by friends and associates, most of whom are our contemporaries. We forget, however, to extend our own thinking to the temporal settings of other people in other age groups, thereby contributing more than our share to generation gaps.

Learning how our older or younger patients use time may be one way to understand and appreciate the differences attributable to other time settings. The saying "An idle mind is the devil's workshop" reflects an attitude prevalent in the early 1900's, when diligent and purposeful use of time was valued, and idleness was not. From such insights, we can begin to see why elderly patients may find it difficult to adjust to retirement and leisure time, or why being in a hospital for a long period may do more psychic harm than the illness.

The slower pace of life in the temporal settings of older persons may also create bewilderment over the rapid pace of today's world. Having to keep up with the times may create frustration and add psychic burdens to their already diminished physical and mental functioning. If time waits for no man, perhaps we can help by adjusting our pace to their speed and understanding of time.

Time as a Sequential Process

Earlier the concept of time was referred to as a temporal dimension that gives sequential order to our lives. Time sequences help us establish the relationship of an event, the behaviors occurring in it, and the time period (consecutive or not) during which both take place.

Time as a sequential process is an essential aspect of our nursing practice. The placement of behaviors and events in time is important in the collection of data for the problem-solving process, which is the basis of our nursing care. Assessing a patient's pain, for example, involves the observation of behaviors indicative of pain, the patient's statement and perception of pain, the duration of it, and the relation of all these factors to the time pain medication was last administered. From these data, decisions can be made either to give additional medication in keeping with the prescribed time sequence or to call the physician for a more effective preparation if the present medication is not helping the patient. The relationship of behavior, event, and time gives perspective to problem-solving endeavors. Time as a sequential process brings together seemingly unrelated facts, events, and behaviors and helps us correlate them into a perspective of cause and effect.

No less important is the sequential process involved in the development of nurse-patient relationships. Each helping relationship and each visit has a beginning, a middle, and an end, but the time sequence of a relationship is the temporal space between visits. These may vary from a visit every day, to weekly, to every second or third week, and may range in time from several weeks to several months and beyond. Short-term relationships, such as in crisis intervention units, involve a limited time sequence as a basis for giving assistance.

Each visit within a relationship builds upon the previous visit. As the time sequence develops, more insight is achieved into the relationship of the patient's behavior, his perception of it, and the events that may have influenced that behavior. Although one visit may reveal some of his concerns and needs, several visits spaced in a sequence of time help give a more complete representation to, and make more valid, our assessments of those concerns and needs. Recurrent themes in a patient's perception, feelings, and behaviors are more likely to be demonstrated during spaced sequential visits than in a single visit. Sequential time weaves these themes together into a pattern and constancy we can understand and use in assisting our patients.

Not all uses of time are orderly in sequence. Several patterns have a suggestion of sequence, but they do not resemble the kind with which we are most familiar — a one-two-three progression. The goal of the sequence is eventually reached, however, because the pattern is arranged with an objective in mind. A circle represents a cyclic sequence, such as the menstrual cycle, during which a woman's body prepares itself for ovulation every twenty-eight to thirty days. Our blood supply undergoes a similar, but very rapid, cycle in order for our tissues to be adequately nourished.

A good deal of security is derived from the sequential element of time, because we can predict, see connections in behavior, build interpersonal relationships, and use it for problem-solving. These and many others bind us solidly to the temporal dimension of the present. For many, however, the security derived from an orderly temporal sequence is often threatened, which then becomes a frightening experience. To the anesthetized patient, time is infinite; there is no beginning, no middle, no end. He may close his eyes, and when he reopens them, hours may have elapsed. All perceptions of day or night or of month or year are lost.

The threat to temporal security can come through use of narcotizing, and to some extent stimulating, drugs. These substances distort time; they may seem to accelerate time, as with stimulants, or suspend it, as with narcotics. Drugs cloud our temporal signposts; there is no real temporal setting, no meaning or value in it, and no sequence. For our patients, awakening after surgery or after a pain medication has worn off, the loss of temporal boundaries, for however short a time, must be frightening. For drug addicts, the suspension of temporal boundaries may be a welcome escape from the restrictions of reality within these units. Regardless of the drugs or treatments involved, we should establish temporal boundaries for all patients through the symbols of time in order that they may experience as much security and orientation as possible while they are in the hospital.

Time as a Measurement of Activity

Nursing care requires time: time to plan, time to implement, and most of all, time to evaluate. The necessity of evaluating our nursing care can never be emphasized enough, because it is the basis for all alterations and improvements. Time provides us with a means of measuring our nursing care in two ways. First, we can determine exactly what nursing tasks have been done within the time assigned to them. Here we use time in a broad sense in order to measure the number or totality of the tasks we have accomplished. Were *all* the medications given? Have *all* my patients received morning care? Did my three patients get back from x-ray? Did Mrs. X. get up in a chair today? These examples describe *what* has been achieved during a certain amount of time.

A second use of time as a measurement is to determine *how* we accomplish our nursing care goals, based on the effectiveness of the nursing tasks we have completed. In this manner, we seek to determine the *quality* of what we have done in the time assigned for it. For example, if all our patients received morning care, *how* was it given? Was it given to conserve the patients' physiological energies? Was it given hastily? Were any observations made or questions asked relative to the patient and his night's sleep? This type of self-examination helps pinpoint our strengths and deficiencies in giving nursing care and allows for a revised approach to our work. Both uses of time help improve the effectiveness of our problem-solving skills and abilities in giving nursing care.

WAITING: ITS USES AND MEANING FOR PATIENTS

For most of our patients, waiting is an important occupation. They have become all too familiar with its demands. Both events and people are the anticipated objects of waiting. Patients wait for the return of their health, for their doctors, for treatment, for someone who cares about them — even death. Each patient reacts differently to waiting and his reactions are communicated to us in a variety of ways that need to be considered.

Waiting as a Human Resource

In a society such as ours that values time so highly, it is not surprising to find a fairly strict adherence to and respect for the observance of time. Punctuality is not only desirable, it is expected. That expectation, however, is tempered by a waiting period built into our individual sense of time and its observance. Within this limit, breeches in punctuality may not result in drastic changes in our temperament; social acceptability is still possible and rationalizations are usually accepted graciously. Beyond this point, however, affability is not always a predominant characteristic of our behavior.

Patients also have a limit for waiting. When we exceed it, we are likely to encounter impatience from them, the degree of which often increases in direct proportion to the length of time beyond their limit for waiting. Frustration, anger, and even open hostility are some of the behavioral outcomes of prolonged or repeated periods of waiting. Impatience is a form of defense expressed in response to what may be considered a cultural insult, and it is not uncommon in patients whose culture highly values the observance and passage of time (and of waiting).

Waiting as Social Meaning

Although impatience and anger may be the behavioral responses to prolonged waiting, the meaning of such expressions needs to be explored. Waiting, as a concept having social meaning, also evokes memories capable of stimulating behaviors and actions in response to a current experience. Loss of self-esteem is one such feeling that is reactivated through waiting. Illness that requires hospitalization has already weakened a patient's self-esteem, and if we make him wait beyond his point of tolerance, we jeopardize it still further. Since actions speak louder than words, particularly with reference to waiting, no amount of verbal persuasion can detract from what a patient has perceived as an indignity. The anxiety produced because of the threat in waiting must be expressed or discharged in order to reduce the discomfort caused by it. The result may be overreaction — expression of more intense behaviors than ordinarily expected in a given situation. Patients may reassert their identities by making additional requests or demands upon us, which in themselves take up our valuable time.

What we communicate to patients, who must endure seemingly endless waiting, is that they as individuals have decreasing worth and that no apparent effort will be made to support their needs for self-esteem. A patient's method of counterattack is defensive behaviors, which at times are his only perceptible means of reaffirming his essential integrity as a human being.

For many patients, waiting has a more serious overtone, stemming from unfulfilled needs for self-esteem, but crystallized by the feeling of abandonment. A patient perceives desertion as a loss of someone or something that has great meaning for him and for which he has great need. Periods of hospitalization intensify these needs. The significance of an object or of people for any one patient is not uniformly perceived as such by others, including ourselves. The value he may assign to objects or to people, therefore, is an important factor in his care, especially if he perceives them as being lost or having left him.

To someone experiencing the stress of hospitalization and a variety of other concerns connected with it, feeling abandoned can be particularly acute. A trachostomy patient, for example, whose life depends on an unclogged airway, may respond to any period of waiting with panic. His need for people he values and depends upon (i.e., ourselves) is paramount, and when his need (in this case, his need for suctioning) does not seem to be met, because his perceptions of time and waiting are distorted by his panic, he feels abandoned — threatened by death if his airway is not patent — left alone — deserted. Likewise, the asthmatic patient whose air supply is threatened sees waiting as a threat to the restoration of his normal breathing.

The suicide of a patient in the hospital activates similar feelings of abandonment in other patients. Would *they* have to wait in vain? Would help come in time? To them, the suicide is the result of our desertion of that patient. Such perceptions may not always be reasonable or justified, but they are not meant to be as long as the threat of abandonment imminently exists in other patients.

An ulcer patient also illustrates the threat of waiting. The dependency needs at the root of his illness reactivate unmet needs of his childhood during periods of what he may consider undue waiting. Each request he makes of us often serves unconsciously to test the dependability of our actions, in addition to reassuring himself that he will not be abandoned through unnecessary waiting.

Waiting implies a sense of power — to control the use of time. In any waiting situation, one person must do the waiting; the person being waited for exerts control by deciding (consciously or not) when to end the waiting period. Persons who exert this kind of control are usually in a position of prestige, authority, or status, which affords them this opportunity. In a hospital, our professional status puts us in such a position of power by virtue of being involved with a variety of time schedules and priorities. We are the ones who very often determine the period of waiting patients must endure. This conveys dominance, although the intent may not be conscious.

In the hospital, the patient must submit to a waiting period decided upon by others, and this leaves him with a feeling of helplessness — a sense of not having control over the situation. This problem is not isolated to time and waiting, but it pertains to all situations in which peoples' control over their lives is reduced. These feelings of helplessness increase when a patient feels that nothing he could say or do would change the events surrounding the use of his time in the act of waiting. Such feelings also communicate futility, and the result is a listless, apathetic patient who expects lengthy periods of waiting, expects to be disappointed if he questions it, and expects no consultation about the use of his time relative to waiting.

Where Waiting Occurs

Settings are temporal spaces designed for the exercise of actions that conclude a period of waiting and result in the achievement of an anticipated event or need. Settings in which waiting occurs are not meant to stifle action or replace it with inaction, yet many of our health settings do just that. Against the backdrops of hospitals, outpatient clinics, and areas within the community, we see self-esteem reduced and feelings of abandonment and helplessness heightened — all playing a part in a patient's frustrating experience of marking time. We are not likely to forget the picture called to mind of patients in these settings — staring faces stamped on tired bodies locked in chairs, primed for the call of their names. Anticipating the event of health care would seem far worse than the reality of it.

Settings in the community also unnecessarily prolong the anticipation of health care. People feel constricted and overpowered by the setting, because it reminds them of needs and serves daily as a reminder of the powerlessness to direct the course of their lives and those of their families. The mother on welfare, whose family is too large for their small apartment, waits daily for word of a new and larger apartment, only to be rewarded with a denial from the social worker. The person from a minority background waits with increasing frustration for the receipt of civil rights guaranteed him in the Constitution. The exertion of control has demonstrated how it is exercised in the use of time and waiting to prolong the expectation of civil rights for some of our citizens.

Settings related to health are varied and the meaning a particular setting has for a patient, together with having to wait for what seems an eternity, can make the atmosphere seem oppressive. This in turn may influence how health care is interpreted. Even the most well-furnished, well-staffed, and clean health care facility can seem oppressive if waiting is followed by dispassionate treatment that is grudgingly administered. Conversely, in mobile health vans and neighborhood health centers constructed from old, unused stores in need of furniture and paint, waiting can be a therapeutic antidote to loneliness if the staff and patients wait *with* each other for the anticipated event of health care.

Waiting as a Sequential Process

The frequency with which waiting occurs in our relationships with patients needs to be carefully observed and evaluated. Not only does it chip away at a patient's self-esteem and evoke defensive communication, but it also soon destroys the trust and rapport of the relationship. A patient may use waiting periodically or consistently to test our investment in him and his welfare. It becomes a method of avoiding involvement for him, often because of the pain of previous relationships. The caring person within a relationship brings the risks of such involvement. The pain of previous involvements often incites an avoidance maneuver in patients who must test the relationship. When these incidents occur, and they do often, they offer us the opportunity to assess the possible cause-and-effect pattern in the patient's behavior.

For us, waiting can provide many opportunities to discover the feelings and reactions we may experience in being left waiting. Identifying the reasons for these emotions, and deciding how to constructively redirect them are additional means of self-discovery. In any one such incident may come new insights we can use in evaluating similar experiences in the future. Through this process we also can better appreciate and understand how a patient must feel in having to wait for hospital or community services.

NURSING CONSIDERATIONS IN THE USE OF TIME AND TIME RELATIONSHIPS

Time is not an unoccupied dimension; we occupy it, use it, and share it with patients. Because their interests are ours, we must discover ways in which time and waiting can be used to better advantage in our nursing practice. Perhaps we need to know not just how we use it but also how we share it with patients.

Sharing time with patients is, admittedly, a luxury. That is not to say that by fulfilling nursing tasks relative to patient care we are not sharing time — we are, but we are sharing it because a task must be done. The time involved with such a task is not wasted; much is gleaned from these moments by both ourselves and patients. Sharing time independent of tasks, procedures, or events means entering the temporal dimension voluntarily (both nurse and patient) in order to establish a supportive coalition to explore what can be done *in* time *with* time, as it is perceived by both participants.

The mutuality in sharing also applies to waiting, because waiting *for* some event or person often is a solitary and uncertain adventure for a patient; being *with* him during a period of waiting indicates the supportive and reassuring aspect of this helping coalition. Such sharing cannot be cultivated in earnest until we determine how it can best be used.

One means at our disposal is to determine how our patients use time and how they tolerate the experience of waiting. Such information, when collected and assessed, can offer us the outline of a plan for nursing action that will involve better utilization of our time together. For example, what are our patients' complaints regarding time and waiting? How frequent are they? Do they come before or after the anticipated event? Is there a relationship between the complaint and the setting in which they wait? How do they cope with the situation? In what ways do they communicate their impatience? Do they press their call lights incessantly? Do they become angry? To whom do they express their impatience and anger? To us? To other patients? To their doctor?

What cultural factors contribute to their frustration with time and waiting? Is the behavior typical for the cultural background as described in nursing and anthropological literature? On the basis of the collected information, what is our nursing approach? Such assessments give us a clearer picture of our patients and their concepts of time and extends our knowledge beyond the immediacy of their illnesses.

Anticipation of an event can be a fearsome prospect for any patient. It can be a lonely situation, because no one can experience what it is like for him. It can be frightening, because he may be waiting for something he does not expect. It may be shattering, because it may bring him news he does not want to hear. Waiting is seldom a compromise between extremes of news for a patient; it is always either good or bad.

Realizing the prospects of waiting faced by many patients, we might best serve their interests by reducing the anticipation. Regardless of how short the waiting period is, it will seem long if nothing fills it and no one shares it.

We can do several things to reduce the anticipation experienced in long periods of waiting. Returning frequently to a patient who must wait is a reassuring gesture, which communicates that he is not being left alone. The same gesture also keeps his temporal boundary within realistic perimeters, even though his concept of time may not be accurate.

Another measure we can utilize is to keep any promises we make with respect to time. Patients rely on our word, and if we say we plan to return in ten minutes, that is when we should be back. Since many patients have difficulty keeping track of time, they need our help in establishing a realistic perception of it. Promises should not be made if they cannot be kept. Unforeseen circumstances do cause even the best intentioned promises to be broken, and when this does happen, patients should have a full explanation for the delay or change in plans. No patient's self-esteem is likely to be elevated by behaviors that communicate he was forgotten.

The unrealistic phrase "I'll be back in a minute" does nothing to help a patient with the realities of time as he experiences it in the hospital. What we are really saying when we use this phrase is "I'll be back when I have time," or "I'll be back if I pass this way again," or "After I finish my work, I'll stop in." Our patients have no way to measure what we mean relative to time in phrases such as these. They need a clear indication of when they can expect us to return, and our promises should be made with consideration for the demands of our schedules and the patient's tolerance for waiting.

Activities of daily living occupy some of a patient's time, but not all of it. If a patient's life style does not include activities of personal interest for him, we can develop them through our nursing care. Many patients do not enjoy reading, for example; others do not enjoy handicrafts, such as knitting and crocheting. For some patients, television is perhaps the only source of enjoyment and stimuli, yet even it is not varied enough to keep them totally occupied.

Interpersonal activities with other patients are an important source of stimuli and support. Aside from the captive audience in a ward situation, there are many other opportunities for socialization that go begging and are not used to advantage. Many elderly patients, tidied and ready for the day ahead, are left to their own devices once their physical care has been completed. Socialization with these patients is an important factor in their ability to relate to others in an appropriate manner. When they are left alone in a hospital or apartment, time, without boundaries, symbols, and people to fill the void, becomes a cruel and exacting tyrant, continually reminding them of each passing minute waiting to be used and shared with someone.

The moments we share with patients, whatever the expectation, fill time with interpersonal closeness and support necessary to lessen whatever threat waiting may pose. The demands upon their personal resources are almost continual during hospitalization. At home they may have few demands for their time, which makes waiting for anything a hollow expectation — one just as stressful. Whatever their past experiences or cultural orientation, they are more than ready for supportive gestures.

Our own efforts to share time with them in waiting must also undergo examination, because we cannot give or share what we do not recognize and understand in ourselves. Knowledge of the social meaning, value, setting, and sequential properties of time and waiting is potentially helpful, but consistent use of problem-solving can link them together into a plan of care that will help ourselves and our patients to understand the experience.

PEOPLE IN COMMUNITIES: SUBJECT TO CHANGE WITHOUT NOTICE

One predominant aspect of our contemporary society is change, not in the planned or gradual sense, but accelerated prolific change. Every day there is increasing evidence of change, which requires more and more adaptation from us. The more rapid change is within our society, the more likely we are to lose contact with what anthropologist Edward Hall calls the "familiar cues" of our cultural system [15]. The phrase *cultural shock* refers to the loss or distortion of familiar cultural cues and their replacement with new ones of another culture, which are less familiar and less comforting to us. In time, however, we have become accustomed to these new cultural cues and have discovered ways to anticipate them or lessen their impact upon us.

The accelerated changes we are currently experiencing in our society leave us with little time for such planning and adaptation. In every facet of human experience we are discovering that our lives are in a perpetual state of change. The cues upon which we have relied within our own culture are no longer dependable or predictable. What once was, remains for a very short time and is no more. As Alvin Toffler proposes in his book *Future Shock,* we experience a "cultural shock within [our] own society" [16]. It emerges, he goes on to say, "as a product of the greatly accelerated rate of change in society . . . [and] arises from the superimposition of a new culture on an old one" [17]. This sudden change and the clashes that occur within us and our society are what Toffler has termed "future shock." He describes it as "the shattering stress and disorientation that we induce in individuals by subjecting them to too much change in too short a time [18].

The future shock Toffler describes with respect to accelerated change has a counterpart in our physical world. For example, pounding waves on a sandy beach and fault lines in the earth's crust constitute the visible results of opposing forces.

> [In our human world] accelerated change . . . is more likely to take place along those interfaces where culture meets culture or different kinds of neighborhoods rub shoulders along a common street. Seen from above, a city is like a mosaic . . . the edges where patterns touch each other are the channels along which change accelerates. In cities, the "dead" areas

are those where borderlines do not exist. Change moves there very slowly. We call them blighted areas. The break boundary in a city may not only be horizontal, as between different neighborhoods, but vertical as in the process of economic and social mobility — layers upon layers with the penthouse on the top. The horror of life in the city slum is an impelling force that motivates the less patient or the more innovative, outward and upward, with the new boundary layers in between each successive stage they attain [19].

As nursing involves us more actively with families of various cultural backgrounds in the community, the evidence of these clashes becomes more apparent. The adjustment encountered by families of any one culture into that of another has become a familiar element in community nursing. Families from the Deep South moving to more urban and industrialized northern cities, for example, must make extensive adjustment to what must seem like a rapid pace of life.

Oriental families newly arrived in the United States from Asian countries are faced with such cultural shocks, because their language virtually isolates them within the linguistic boundaries of their culturally similar but new community. From a homeland where obedience and loyalty are important aspects of family life, they are faced with the relaxation of these concepts by Oriental families in their newly adopted home. These are some changes of which we have become aware and for which we have tried to prepare.

The behaviors and attitudes expressive of the accelerated change within our society are becoming increasingly apparent. When we visit families in various neighborhoods within the community, we see that they are often unable to understand and keep abreast of events. Problems of adaptation may arise because the change was unexpected or the family does not have a plan for constructive adaptation to it. The problem is not necessarily the change, because change has become inevitable, but the ability of the family and its members to cope with it through constructive and flexible adaptation.

CHANGE AS A COMMUNICATED BEHAVIOR

As we become professionally more active in the community and learn to develop our communication skills effectively, we become more aware of the relation of our families' communication to the accelerated changes within society. Communication as an expression of such change may take many forms and often be explosive. People may exhibit anger, frustration, depression, apathy, antagonism, violence (verbal or physical), or behaviors directed against a neighborhood, the community, and its institutions.

For many of us the expression of these behaviors is a professional shock, because so much of the behaviors we have become accustomed to have been confined within the boundaries of our professional culture, such as hospitals and clinics. Here, with the exception of psychiatric wards, the communicated behaviors of our patients are generally predictable and within the expectations of those boundaries.

Families within the community, however, are not as easily categorized or understood. Our presence alone may represent more than just an attempt to communicate interpersonally; it may symbolize either the elements of society that have inflicted the changes with which they feel unable to cope or the elements that have prevented change from progressing fast enough. Our interpersonal communication at these times may not be as much between two people, or between nurse and family, as between two seemingly opposing cultures, in which the forces and pressures of change are interpreted and responded to in different and often conflicting ways. Such was the case in the following example:

> A group of nursing students had invited 25 elderly people for a tour of the campus. They had been visiting the elderly in their homes and wished to return the hospitality they had been shown. During the coffee hour following the tour, a nursing student noticed that an 85-year-old black lady, Mrs. A., had not removed her coat. She approached the lady and asked if she would like to check her wrap in the adjoining room. The woman declined. Several other students, not aware that the woman had been approached, offered the same assistance and were given the same answer. The room was not cold, and all of the other guests (including other black ladies) had removed their coats, so it was mystifying for the students to see one person firmly wishing to wear hers.
>
> A few days after the event, the students and their instructor met for a conference, and discussion focused on the behavior of Mrs. A. A few students felt it was "weird," and others found it puzzling and wondered what it had meant. They asked the student who was visiting her to explore the matter further.
>
> Several weeks later when another conference was held, the nursing student shared her findings with the group. In the time that had lapsed, she had talked with the volunteers (both black and white) at the senior centers the lady attended as well as with Mrs. A. Her information shed light on the behavior the students had observed.
>
> Mrs. A. was raised in the Deep South, where segregation was strictly enforced. Lapses in this way of life often meant humiliation or punishment, so Mrs. A. was taught always to be careful. Her life style provided that she was always separate from whites, and separation included one's coats in the cloakroom. At the senior center, Mrs. A. regularly sat and wove at a loom nearest the door and kept her coat on. One of the volunteers remembered that her own mother used to wear her wrap all the time, because, in case there was any trouble, she could leave fast without having to find it.
>
> Mrs. A. remarked that integration was good, but it was for the young. She said, "I can't keep up with all these changes. It seems like all of a sudden everything happened and suddenly I'm equal with them. Well that isn't my way. I don't feel equal just because they're tellin' me I am.

I've been taught differently, and gettin' chummy with whites just isn't my way. I can't forget 85 years of being unequal; I can't change now — I won't change now."

With this information, the students began to understand how difficult it must be for Mrs. A. to change a lifetime of behavior to accommodate the rapid changes integration had brought.

One behavioral attitude that many of us communicate to our patients and families is the belief that our culture is superior to all others. This is called ethnocentric behavior, and implicit in it is the attitude that other people should be like us regardless of their cultural orientation. For this we earned the title of "Ugly American" from our European and Asian allies in World War II. Another example on a larger, more tragic scale was Adolph Hitler's Third Reich. The belief in Aryan superiority and the need to keep Aryan stock free from contamination by cultural inferiors resulted in the death of six million Jews in a government program of racial genocide.

Today we are experiencing many forms of social change and upheaval as various cultural groups within our neighborhoods, communities, and country struggle for identity, civil and social equality, and recognition as fully participating members of society. Years of seeing civil rights, justice, housing, and equal job opportunities ignored, delayed, and compromised have produced a seemingly sudden demand for change. Around us we see blacks, American Indians, Chicanos, and Orientals steadily and more confidently exercising their cultural voices in the conduct of our society.

Interactions between ourselves and families can be difficult at best if we retain an ethnocentric disposition. We often are so intent on our nursing task that we fail to be aware that the communication of families is part of a cultural pattern, and the means by which frustration with sociocultural change and adaptation are expressed. When the term *racist* is hurled at us, for example, it is personally offensive, particularly if we do not understand that it represents the exasperation of one culture for another that does not acknowledge a different cultural background.

Visiting families and traveling are good ways to learn about other cultures — to be open to new ideas and people — thereby reducing the ethnocentric fervor of our attitudes and behavior. Even so, there is no assurance that our efforts will not be met with suspicion and cynicism. To people of other cultural backgrounds, we, with our naive attempts to become culturally enlightened, have been preceded by many others whose enthusiasm faltered and whose promises never materialized. The challenge, either spoken or unspoken, becomes clear when we are faced with it: "What makes you think you're any different from all the others?" · Such a challenge forces us to acknowledge the reality of the situation and to supply an answer.

Not all of us may be able to give an open, honest, and believable answer; some of us may not want to supply one. In such a confrontation, as professional nurses, we should keep in mind that the United States, as the melting pot, is comprised of various ingredients, each of which has a distinct flavor that adds something different and special to the substance being cooked. It would be a shame for us to see and taste the dish without inquiring into the recipe. Ethnocentrism is like cooking a dish with only one ingredient, the results are unpalatable and bound to cause cultural malnourishment. The challenge we are faced with every day from families in the community is that we have been cooking on one burner with one ingredient for too long.

ADAPTATION TO CHANGE

The anticipation of change poses a severe threat to the security of long-held values, beliefs, attitudes, and feelings. Until now they have proved predictable, expedient, and useful in our conduct of life. With change, we are also faced with the necessity of exchanging our base of security for something that is unknown and unpredictable, and whose rewards are, at the very least, uncertain. Present gains seem far more appealing than those we may achieve in the future. Change, therefore, has an attendant uncertainty — not only in rewards, but also in our ability to adapt to it.

These doubts may bring to mind our weaknesses and vulnerabilities; they may precipitate failure in adapting to changes or remind us of past failures to do so. Also present is the fear of losing the rewards we have already achieved.

As these changes become more rapid, unanticipated, and numerous, our ability to adapt may be impaired and the effects on us may be more visible. Each human being, as an adaptive organism among similar organisms, experiences the same urgency and need to succeed, despite the nature of the change, and all wish to succeed with the same goal in mind. The noted psychiatrist Dr. Karl Menninger describes this goal as:

> ... trying to survive, with minimal pain and maximal pleasure, including the pleasures of achievement, of pride, and of loyalty to principle. All of this requires an infinitude of doing, of trying and failing, of trying and succeeding and having to compromise. It involves going ahead, stepping aside, stepping back, perhaps even running away. It involves fights and embraces, bargains and donations, gestures and conversations, working and playing, reproaches, rewards and retrenchments.
>
> This is the uncomplicated process of living, with all major contingencies, including those of growing older and feebler, temporarily left out of consideration. But, as we all know there are contingencies. The unexpected is always happening. Emergencies are constantly arising. The "mis"-behavior of other individuals, the occurrence of disruptive events, the change in certain situations — deaths, births, accidents — all sorts of

things happen which may strain the capacity of the individual for easy accommodation. His comfort, his gratifications, perhaps even his growth or safety are threatened. Such a challenge stimulates extra or renewed effort, and he puts up the best battle he can for the best possible bargain under the changed circumstances of the new situation [20].

The best possible bargain is not always available during accelerated or severe change. Recent scientific investigation has shown that the more we are faced with severe changes, the more we are likely to succumb to marked physiological, psychological, and environmental stresses. These studies point to the growing need for all of us to focus our attention on the way our patients and families in the community adapt to the bombardment of accelerated changes in everyday living. Toffler poses a question for consideration in our interactions with families. He asks, "By studying the amount of change in a person's life, could we learn anything about the influence of change itself on health" [21]? The answer seems obvious.

The continuity of our visits, together with spatial proximity and psychological closeness, gives us ideal opportunities to observe how a family and its members cope with everyday stresses. From our visits we begin to learn and to understand a family, its history, its tasks and problems of growth and development, and the emerging changes in perspective it brings. By identifying patterns of daily adaptation, we gain information basic to the intuitive problem-solving behavior of each family and individual in it. These patterns are predictable, and can indicate resilience and flexibility, depending on the degree of adaptation.

When a family or one of its members is unable to successfully use familiar means of adapting or coping, a crisis exists. In such situations, which may be threatening to life, growth, or safety, new resources must be found and new behaviors tested in order to achieve the "best possible bargain" in the face of the impending threat. We must alert ourselves to the kinds of behaviors within a family that establish its pattern of adaptation.

Crises require immediate attention, and we can easily lose sight of a family's normative patterns of coping and the success they have achieved in dealing with their problems. Instead of building on the potential strengths already demonstrated, and which may have important sociocultural implications, we often offer our assistance as if such behaviors were nonexistent or unproductive. The family's potentials for health are never really explored or utilized if earlier patterns of coping are not examined and channeled in a positive direction. In times of social crisis, a family's receptivity for help is often greater; their potential for change and their willingness to activate it are also greater.

Mobilizing that potential is the problem of all of us, who as professionals see the complexities of family life in urban areas multiply — demanding increasingly more adaptation than one family can make. Psychiatrist Leonard Duhl expresses this problem and what he feels is the responsibility of health professionals in this matter:

> I am concerned about change and that we psychiatrists [nurses and others] apply some of our knowledge of its processes to the problems of the city and of the alienated. We do not really know what makes the city work. I am quite convinced now, there is nobody who really understands how fantastically complex this living organism known as a city is. We must all begin to learn about it . . . by total immersion. We've got to get in it, to see it, and smell it and feel it.
>
> The city is made up of a thousand micro-cities. And if you are trying to learn the whole of the city and how it operates as a total organism, you have to find out what each micro-city is and how all the pieces and parts fit together.
>
> *To do that,* we should learn together, not only because it is easier, but because we must learn each other's language so we can talk the same game. I think the hardest problem I had was to speak English. I speak "psychiatrist-ese" and everybody expects me to do it. Many of the psychiatrists I know who are interested in the city and are working with people concerned with urban problems also speak "psychiatrist-ese". And nobody else understands what they are talking about.
>
> . . . The critical problem is to maintain communications, to keep the avenues of communication open; because as the loss of communication and polarization grows, the possibility of solution diminishes. We all know this principle works also in terms of [the] family [unit and its] welfare: the minute communication stops, family unity begins to deteriorate. I am concerned because the temptation seems everywhere to be finding ways of increasing the polarization [22].

The demands made upon us because of rapid and multiple changes within our society affect each of us by determining the patterns of our behavioral response and by "contributing to the shaping of our personalities by interfering with the acquisition of new experiences" [23].

It remains for us to immerse ourselves in the communities where we live and work in order to learn how families think, feel, and act, because here, at the interfaces of our human world, the opposing forces will clash — the immovable force of the *haves* against the struggling, convulsive movement of the *have nots*. These human forces will determine our future and our ability to accept and adapt constructively to change. The determinants are in each family unit. Those potentials can be tapped, but only if we understand and learn what is involved in the process of change and its effect on the adaptive abilities of a family and its members.

SUMMARY

Every facet of our lives is influenced by our sociocultural background. Territoriality, privacy, time, waiting, and change represent a small part of that influence, but one full of meaning as we meet, interact, and learn about the people we expect to help. Regardless of who they are, where they are, or their background, we will be affected by them. The circumstances of illness and the potentials for health are no less influential and are related directly to each person's sociocultural background. We, therefore, must learn even more about how these backgrounds affect the quality of our nursing care.

Some sociocultural principles that can be applied to our nursing care are as follows:

1. Each culture is of primary importance to its possessor and is reflected through interpersonal behavior.

2. Knowledge of the ways each individual has been influenced by his culture allows us to predict certain aspects of present and future behavior.

3. "One can be physically and geographically in a culture and yet not psychologically in it" [24].

4. Spatial proximity determines the quality of communication necessary in a helping relationship.

5. The function of privacy is protective — to insure the development and preservation of our individuality.

6. Increased sensory input requires that privacy be maintained either spatially or psychologically for requisite amounts of time by every human being in order to maintain emotional equilibrium.

7. Time is a temporal boundary within space, which gives our behavior order and meaning.

8. Consistent use of the symbols of time provides reality as well as order for our patients.

9. Periods of waiting that extend beyond one's inner time limit can precipitate defensive communication.

10. One's response to change and its rewards is determined by the degree, the rate, and the meaning of the change.

NOTES

1. Hall, Edward T. *The Silent Language,* pp. 31—41.
2. Ardrey, Robert. *The Territorial Imperative,* p. 3.
3. Barnlund, Dean. *Interpersonal Communication: Survey and Studies,* pp. 515—516.
4. Hall, Edward. *The Hidden Dimension,* p. 45.
5. Ibid., pp. 113—125.
6. Bloch, Dorothy W. *Behavioral Concepts and Nursing Interventions,* pp. 253—254.
7. Tillich, Paul. *The Eternal Now,* pp. 17—18.
8. Schwartz, Barry. The Social Psychology of Privacy, p. 743.

9. Ibid., p. 243.
10. Hayakawa, S. I. *Modern Guide to Synonyms,* p. 150.
11. Hoggart, Richard. *The Uses of Literacy,* p. 62.
12. Merwin, William S. *The Carrier of Ladders,* p. 15.
13. Hoggart, op. cit. (note 11), p. 62.
14. Clarke, Arthur C. The Tyranny of Time, p. 81.
15. Hall, op. cit. (note 1), p. 156.
16. Toffler, Alvin. *Future Shock,* p. 11.
17. Ibid., p. 11.
18. Ibid., p. 2.
19. Kaiser Aluminum News, *The Dynamics of Change,* p. 16.
20. Menninger, Karl. *The Vital Balance,* pp. 126–127.
21. Toffler, op. cit. (note 16), p. 329.
22. Duhl, Leonard. *Distress in the City,* pp. 115–118.
23. Dubos, René. *Man, Medicine and Environment,* p. 41.
24. Fenalason, Anne F. *Essentials in Interviewing: For the Interviewer Offering Professional Services,* p. 49.

BIBLIOGRAPHY

Ardrey, Robert. *The Territorial Imperative.* New York: Atheneum, 1966.
Barnlund, Dean. *Interpersonal Communication: Survey and Studies.* Boston: Houghton Mifflin, 1968.
Bennis, Warren G., Benne, Kenneth, and Chin, Robert, eds. *The Planning of Change.* New York: Holt, Rinehart and Winston, 1961.
Bloch, Dorothy W. Privacy. In Carolyn E. Carlson, coordinator. *Behavioral Concepts and Nursing Interventions.* Philadelphia: Lippincott, 1970.
Boeth, Richard. The Assault on Privacy. *Newsweek,* 76:15, 1970.
Clarke, Arthur C. The Tyranny of Time. *Horizon,* 4:80, July, 1962.
Dubos, René. *Man, Medicine and Environment.* New York: Praeger, 1968.
Duhl, Leonard. Psychiatry and the Urban Poor. In William Ryan, ed. *Distress in the City.* Cleveland: Press of Case Western Reserve University, 1969.
Fenalason, Anne E. *Essentials in Interview: For the Interviewer Offering Professional Services.* New York: Harper, 1952.
Hall, Edward T. *The Hidden Dimension.* Garden City, N.Y.: Doubleday, 1969.
Hall, Edward T. *The Silent Language.* Greenwich, Conn.: Fawcett, 1959.
Hayakawa, S. I. *Modern Guide to Synonyms.* New York: Funk & Wagnalls, 1968.
Heirich, Max. The Use of Time in the Study of Social Change. *American Sociological Review,* 29:386, 1964.
Hoggart, Richard. *The Uses of Literacy.* Fairlawn, N.J.: Essential Books, 1957.
Kaiser Aluminum News. *The Dynamics of Change.* Oakland, Calif: Kaiser Aluminum and Chemical Corp., 1966.
Kantor, Mildred, ed. *Mobility and Mental Health.* Springfield, Ill.: Thomas, 1965.
Kastenbaum, Robert. As the Clock Runs Out. *Mental Hygiene,* 50:332, July, 1966.
Merwin, William S. "Words from a Totem Animal." In *The Carrier of Ladders.* New York: Atheneum, 1970.
Moore, Wilbert F. *Man, Time and Society.* New York: Wiley, 1963.

Parks, Suzanne L. Allowing Physical Distance as a Nursing Approach. *Perspectives in Psychiatric Care*, 4:31, 1966.

Pluckhan, Margaret L. Space: The Silent Language. *Nursing Forum*, 7:386, 1968.

Proshansky, Harold M., Ittelson, William H., and Rivlin, Leanne G. *Environmental Psychology: Man and His Physical Setting*. New York: Holt, Rinehart and Winston, 1970.

Roth, Julius A., *Timetables*. Indianapolis: Bobbs-Merrill, 1963.

Sawry, James and Telford, Charles. *Dynamics of Mental Health: The Psychology of Adjustment*. Boston: Allyn & Bacon, 1964.

Schwartz, Barry. The Social Psychology of Privacy. *American Journal of Sociology*, 73:741, 1967–1968.

Smoyak, Shirley. Cultural Incongruence: The Effect on Nurses Perception. *Nursing Forum*, 7:234, 1968.

Tillich, Paul. *The Eternal Now*. New York: Schribner, 1963.

Toffler, Alvin. *Future Shock*. New York: Random House, 1970.

IV

Messages

9

The Criteria for Sending Effective Messages

THE WORDS EXCHANGED between human beings are like rich tapestries, woven into varied and colorful patterns with the threads of human thought, feeling, and experience. Each thread is linked to the pattern, and the way each is used in the design influences the tone or brilliance of the color. As tapestries portray an event or person, words also represent ideas and events that need to be shared and exchanged between people.

Words are fashioned by man to convey his meaning, articulate his ideas, and transmit his perceptions. Because human language provides such limitless creativity, man can use words to speak of things remembered or imagined, of things abstract or concrete, and of things simple or complex. Every time man uses words, he demonstrates his capacity for creativity — of coining new words or phrases, inviting new ideas, and posing new questions — which adds to his ability to perceive and understand the people and events surrounding him.

As he becomes inventive with language and uses it in a structured form recognized by others, man becomes better able to "identify, objectify, describe, standardize, classify and universalize all [his] different types of experience" [1]. These elaborative tasks require variety that invokes his curiosity and ingenuity in the exploration of ways words can be used in our language. Such exploration is not an impulsive escapade, because it is essential that man be understood. For comprehension to take place, we must exercise, with selectivity, the formulation of words that, when structured in a logical, orderly manner, clearly and effectively convey our message. Such efforts link our perceptions of different experiences and the person to whom we are talking.

The richness of our language invites countless possibilities in the exchange of information between ourselves and patients, which need not be confined to the problems of illness, but can extend into all areas in which our patients express their concern and interest. Just as communication in general requires order and choice for people to understand each other, so too does the act of communicating with patients require careful selection of words and deliberation on how they can and should be used.

Whether we refer to an orderly sequence of words (i.e., message code), of what we have to say (i.e., message content) through them, or of how we plan to use them (i.e., message treatment), the effectiveness of our communication with patients is directly related to the way we plan and present our messages. In determining the effectiveness of the choice and use of our messages, several criteria must be considered: efficiency, appropriateness, flexibility, and feed-back* [2]. Each has a direct relation to the coding, content, and treatment of the messages we send to patients.

EFFICIENCY

An efficient message is a clear message. It is concise, constructed simply, and well-timed in that the patient has an opportunity to absorb, reflect, and respond to it. Efficiency in effectively communicating with patients is deceptive. A simple message can become lost in the complexities of language, in the inability to adjust our vocabulary, and in our impatience to achieve a response or goal. All these factors adversely influence the coding or orderly sequence of our message.

Simplicity, clarity, and timing — these are the components of an efficient message that we need to examine further. There is an abundance of words in our language from which to select and frame our messages. Diversity is possible not only because of the richness of our language, but also because of the variety of patients with whom we interact. Their cultural backgrounds, knowledge, and education determine their levels of understanding and their level of vocabulary skills and abilities.

Our professional world involves complex, technical language, which often is impossible for even the most informed layman to understand. In time, we become accustomed to the sound of it and treat it as casually as we would any other natural event. We soon discover, however, that this can be a communication barrier in our interactions with patients, because they do not understand the message we are trying to convey.

Simplicity of language is emphasized here because effort is required to intentionally select simple words to express our message to others. It is far easier to

*Feedback will be discussed in a separate section of this book.

use bigger words because they generally define themselves. Words such as hyperplasia, hypoglycemia, and cholecystectomy are explicit, and we therefore, often assume that they are as clear to others as they are to us. Take the following example: "Coruscate, coruscate diminutive stellar orb; how inexplicable to me is the stupendous problem of your existence." In simpler terms it means: "Twinkle, twinkle, little star, how I wonder what you are." When we use inefficient ways of conveying a message, we must stop, retrace our communication, and begin again, hopefully with simpler words. This increases the interpersonal comfort of patients. Such was the case in the following example:

> The doctor and the head nurse visited his patient, Mrs. C., in order to explain the nature of her illness. "Your tests have indicated that you have diabetes," the doctor began. "This means your pancreatic metabolism is impaired in its ability to manufacture insulin and therefore your digestive processes cannot utilize the glucose you ingest. As a result, your body excretes the unused glucose. We will try to restore some balance to your system by supplying the insulin needed to utilize your intake of glucose." After a few more minutes of explanation the doctor left the room and a confused Mrs. C.

Let us consider the message sent by the doctor. Certainly its coding process indicates a good selection of words in orderly sequence. It was explicit and informative. The only problem was that the patient did not understand what the doctor was trying to tell her. The message he sent was inefficient because the vocabulary used to code it was too complex and the information was lost.

The problem of trying to simplify the language of our messages also points to the need for clarity. If something is not understood by another person, it is not clear. The Roman rhetorician Quintilian once remarked, "One should not aim at being possible to understand, but at being impossible to misunderstand" [3]. To do this we need to make consistent use of the broad selection available in our vocabularies. The doctor in the example had a good vocabulary, but he did not exercise selectivity in making clear what he wanted to say to a person outside his professional circle.

Careful observation of how our messages are being received nonverbally by patients can also assist us in making any necessary adjustments in our coding process. Clarity can be achieved if we keep our messages free of repetition, awkardness, and excessive detail.

In addition to simplicity and clarity is the factor of proper timing. Patients must be allowed sufficient opportunity to absorb the message and respond to it with some measure of feedback. Let us continue with Mrs. C. and the information she received from her doctor.

> After the doctor left the room, Mrs. C. looked confused and said to the nurse, who remained behind, "Just what *did* he say other than I have

diabetes? He lost me after that." The head nurse replied that the doctor had been trying to explain what diabetes was and what he planned to do to help her.

"Well, it certainly sounded impressive," said Mrs. C., "but I'd be just as content if it sounded clearer. Could you do the honors and try explaining it to me again?"

"Certainly," responded the nurse. "Diabetes is a condition that results when an organ in your body called the pancreas is not able to manufacture insulin, which is important because it helps use up the sugar you eat. Without insulin present in adequate amounts, your body cannot handle all the sugar you eat daily. Your body, therefore, has to get rid of the excess. So the extra sugar is released through your system. Testing your urine is one way of telling whether you might have diabetes. What the doctor plans to do for you is to supply your body with the insulin it needs so that the sugar you eat will be used up and not wasted. Insulin is given by injection. Your doctor will decide the amount you need."

Looking relieved, Mrs. C. made a final comment, "So why didn't he say that in the first place!"

In this instance we can see that Mrs. C. not only was more than ready to listen to what the head nurse had to say, but she also indicated that this was the best time to convey a clearer, simpler message.

Despite the extensive number of words in the English language (about 600,000 and still increasing), the number we use in everyday conversation remains pitifully small (about 2000). Many of those we do employ have multiple uses, implying a variety of meanings. (For example, there are approximately 832 ways the word *run* can be used.) Considering that each patient we meet has experiences, capabilities, vocabulary, and knowledge different from all other patients, our ability to construct efficient messages is often tested. What we need is more practice in selecting, from the variety of words possible, those that convey a simple, clear, and well-timed message. With this in mind we may come nearer to our aim; to be impossible to be misunderstood.

APPROPRIATENESS

While the efficiency of a message concerns the way we select and structure our words, its appropriateness concerns the pertinence of those words to the situation at hand. No amount of selectivity will help us if what we say has no application — no relation to the patient and his problem or concern. Misinterpretations are apt to occur if the message we are trying to convey makes little sense, and there are several reasons for them. First, the patient may be receiving more information than can be comfortably absorbed and answered. This is called overloading. Second, a patient may not be getting enough information so that he can respond intelligently. This is called underloading. Finally, we may not be saying what we mean. This is called incongruency. These three factors are much like circuit breakers in a patient's sequential processes of thought and communication. The more these processes are interrupted, the more likely a patient will become confused or inhibited.

Overloading a patient with more information than he needs or is pertinent is a common pitfall in nursing, especially if both the patient and the situation are new to us. Talking too much or engaging in irrelevant verbiage provides us with a way of relieving whatever anxiety we may be experiencing at the time. There is comfort in this, but it must not be the overriding priority in planning our responses. Not only does overloading bombard a patient with verbiage, but it also submerges him in meanings and information he may not be equipped to handle. It places a burden of responsibility on him that he may not wish to assume — responsibility for the things we may inadvertently be sharing with him. Patients may sense our insecurity and anxieties, and they may be made to feel unnecessarily apprehensive about having us involved in their care.

A patient can be bombarded with information in a variety of ways: by being overtalkative when supplying information, asking multiple questions in the same breath, discussing irrelevancies, or pushing him to talk about a topic he may not be ready to discuss. Whatever the method of overloading, the outcome remains the same — reciprocal communication becomes temporarily blocked. The following example illustrates this point. The nurse was beginning to initiate a therapeutic relationship with Mrs. K., a middle-aged woman, who was aloof and distrustful. In this interview, the nurse planned to explain the purpose of her visits to Mrs. K.:

> *Nurse:* When I first told you that I would be seeing you until December, I'm not sure that I made things very clear, and so I would like to clarify them today. Do you know why we talk with each other every day? [I was afraid of sounding too devious — I was interested in her, yet I didn't know what to say.]
>
> *Mrs. K.:* No. Not exactly. [She seemed to be staring at me intently. Her posture was rigid.]
>
> *Nurse:* Well, let me see how to explain it. We're talking together because I like you and am interested in you and want to work with you. But there's more to it than that. It has two main purposes. You are helping me to learn how to talk with other people, but more important, this is your time to talk about anything that you want. You can talk about any problems you have or what's going on around here; or you don't have to talk about anything. By talking together perhaps we can solve some problems and understand things better. If nothing else, I can just listen and be a sounding board for you and help clarify some questions for you. We can also carry some requests that you may have to the proper people. Answer questions. Many things. [Silence. Mrs. K. stared to one side of me with folded hands and pursed lips.]

> *Nurse:* Well, I just wanted to tell you these things and clear things up, since I hadn't been very clear before. I will be coming to see you every day, once in the morning when you come back from work and again in the afternoon. We can sit wherever you like. Remember this is your time to say what you want — to discuss your feelings, thoughts, and any problems you may have. I will listen and help you, and the two of us together may clarify some things. Do you have any questions? How do you feel about this?
>
> *Mrs. K.:* No. [Silence. She stared at the floor for about three minutes.]

In this interaction the nurse, in her uncertainty and anxiety, overwhelmed the patient with a barrage of information, which did nothing to invite the patient's response. It also conveyed messages that could easily be misconstrued, namely, the intent of the nurse to be a listener and to allow the patient to talk.

Asking too many questions in too short a space of time or consecutively without pause is another way of overloading patients, as we see in the following example:

> Miss S. was visiting Mrs. H., an elderly widow living in an older section of the city. During one of the visits, Mrs. H. asked Miss S. if she would like to see the rest of the house. Miss S. eagerly accepted. After the tour, Miss S. in her enthusiasm, began to inquire about several aspects of the house she had found interesting. "How long have you lived in this house? Were you and your husband the original owners or had other people been here before you? Your furniture is so lovely. In fact, these pieces look like antiques. Are they?"

Knowing which question to answer first can be a dilemma for anyone. Many times, without thinking, we place similar expectations on patients and wonder why they may seem momentarily bewildered. Regardless of the number of questions we may have, we can facilitate better responses from our patient if we ask one at a time, giving him time to respond to each one. In this way we clearly establish the focus and priority of our inquiries.

Discussing irrelevancies is another means of injecting inappropriate content into the interview. Such digressions are similar to those of a child whose attention is distracted by a sudden movement or the color of a toy. The fact that the child is eating fades in importance momentarily until the distraction loses its appeal.

In settings in which we interact with patients, there are many distractions and many topics that may be tempting to pursue. At times, in our eagerness to gain needed information, we unwittingly crowd a patient with questions about topics that he may not be ready to discuss. Our curiosity, requiring satisfaction, is the personal need we must satisfy, and in doing so we forget how threatening it can be for him. Talking about death to a patient who has a terminal illness and is unable to face the reality of it, or asking an alcoholic why he drinks to excess and denies it at the same time, illustrates what can happen when we lose sight of whose needs we are supposed to be meeting. In light of that, we must examine ourselves and our motives carefully to discover why such actions are so important to us.

Messages that have inadequate content give our patient very little opportunity to respond intelligently. It then becomes his responsibility, in a sense, to ferret out the content he needs for a proper response. The alternative is to make assumptions, which almost never leads to a satisfactory response and is of little benefit in patient care. Receiving messages with consistently insufficient content is frustrating for someone who already feels under stress, because it does not provide adequate stimulation in a communication exchange. Without practice, patients can gradually lose their verbal elasticity. Several Americans who were recently released from the People's Republic of China after having been imprisoned for several years commented on their difficulties in speaking English fluently. During their imprisonment they had little or no contact with English-speaking people, and minimal English had been spoken.

Habitual use of cryptic or monosyllabic responses creates difficulty and confusion in patients who may need the reassurance of an explanation, the support of a sentence or two, or the encouragement of a pertinent question.

Saying what we mean and meaning what we say — this is called congruency. It is a partnership of words and behavior that match — that go together — that fit like two spoons of a matched set. Congruency means that "we are unified and whole all the way through; our primary experience (including our basic sensations, impulses, desires and needs), our concise awareness and our overt communication are essentially consistent" [4].

Words without their nonverbal components are only half the message — like a melody played without orchestration; we hear the tune, but not the harmony. Because our nonverbal behavior is not totally under our conscious control, we are less apt to know how it affects our words — the tune. In this respect, "words become the shadows of actions" [5]. They are the outline, but without the detail or shades of meaning that are conveyed more accurately through our actions.

All of us differ in our ability to be congruent when we convey our messages, just as we differ in our sensitivity to different types of communication. Some of us ignore much of what we hear, but are extraordinarily sensitive to nonverbal communication. Others prefer to take what a person says verbally as the whole message. Either way, selectivity diverts us from receiving a message as it was intended, namely, with verbal and nonverbal components.

The either-or quality in this kind of communication can be hazardous in nursing. When our communication is incongruent, it confuses a patient as to which of our messages he should respond. This creates doubt. Which messages should he believe? He begins to suspect our intentions and mistrust our interest in his welfare. Our insensitivity to his predicament compounds the problem.

Incongruent messages, unfortunately, proliferate in our encounters with patients. The following incidents serve as examples:

> A group of nursing students was being given a tour of the hospital unit where they would begin their learning experience. During the tour, an adolescent female patient dashed up to one of them and exclaimed with enthusiasm, "I can hardly wait for you to begin. How exciting!"
>
> Visibly startled, the student stiffened noticeably, yet managed to respond politely that he was glad to be starting, too.
>
> The patient then said, "I didn't frighten you did I?"
>
> "Oh no", said the student, "not at all."

> A patient who was recovering from major surgery was worried about his ability to take care of himself at home. He had heard people talk about all the problems a person can have at home and wondered if he would be plagued with them, too. After his morning care, he asked his nurse if she had some time to talk with him about his concerns. She remarked that she did have time and would be glad to help him. As the patient began to discuss his worries, he noticed that the nurse periodically looked at her watch. Though she attempted to be attentive, the patient began to lose interest in continuing to express himself. Shortly thereafter, he said, "Oh well, I guess things will turn out all right." The nurse agreed with him and left the room, wondering why the patient had ended the conversation so soon after it had begun.

Being congruent in our communication means relinquishing pretense — of saying things and acting in ways that do not mean what we want them to mean. Congruency requires practice — practice in observing those of our co-workers who are congruent in their daily interactions with patients and then using our own communication style in a way that coordinates what we mean with what we say. This should not be confused with being bluntly honest. There is no advantage in undiplomatically pointing out to a patient the deficiencies we may see in his personality.

The more we can achieve congruency in our communication, the more we become real, dependable people to our patients. *We* are the only ones who can demonstrate those qualities. As we become better able to match what we say with what we mean, our patients begin to trust us with *themselves* and the things they want and need to share with us. Is this not what we want them to do?

FLEXIBILITY

Regardless of how efficiently or appropriately we arrange our message, its implementation is dependent upon the person for whom it is intended. Because we cannot always be sure how our message will be received, we must consider a third criterion — flexibility. In a previous chapter, the treatment of a message was specified as the decisions we make about the selection and arrangement of the code and content. Decisions made relative to what we say and how we say it must include consideration for the receiver — our patient, his personality, communication style, sociocultural background, and all other qualities that distinguish him as an individual. Since each patient is unique, changing, and different from all others in both perceptions and experiences, it is unlikely that we will encounter another whose everyday communicative behavior is the same.

Good days, bad days, and busy days *all* affect our communication and, in turn, affect others. Because we cannot expect a person's behavior to be unchangeable, flexibility is necessary. Flexibility is an adaptive maneuver that enables us to alter our message with respect to whatever behavioral clue a patient may send. Being flexible means that the response we choose should not be grounded in extremes. In other words, our messages should not be so automatic that we give the impression we are unconcerned or so controlled that little information is exchanged. Both extremes increase the likelihood of inhibiting responses. Considering the importance of what the patient may have to contribute, this can mean an appreciable loss of data.

The ability to be flexible is based on observation of the cues a patient transmits in our presence. They are distinctive of a behavioral "signature" and influence what we say to him and how we say it.

Since helping communication presumes a goal that is centered on the patient or client, it is often difficult to be flexible without feeling that we have deserted the goal that has been so carefully planned. Opportunities to pursue patient-centered goals can be built into preplanned communication. Many more opportunities occur, however, which cannot be anticipated and require keen sensitivity and observation to be noticed and used. When a preplanned goal conflicts with a more immediate one, we must remember to ask ourselves, "Which is more important, meeting the goal *I* have planned or responding to the cues (and therefore the needs) I now perceive my patient to be sending?" Often this struggle occurs when a patient's need is the greatest, as illustrated by the nurse in the following incident:

> I arranged to meet Mrs. B. today after her doctor's appointment at the shopping center. From there I could drive her home and visit awhile with her before I returned to campus for a class. My plan was to explore how she liked her new neighborhood now that she had a new apartment and how it differed from her previous neighborhood. I felt she might be experiencing adjustment problems. It was a nice feeling to have a goal in mind, considering that I had nothing special in mind last time.
>
> When I met Mrs. B., she suggested that we stop for some tea because she hadn't had breakfast yet. (It was 11 a.m. I will have to look into this.) As we had tea, Mrs. B. seemed eager to talk and finally said, "Do you know what I found out yesterday?" She did not wait for me to

answer, but continued, "I found out from a friend that my son's wife had another baby two months ago, and they never wrote to let me know about it. I guess *I know* where *I* stand. Nobody is interested in grandmothers these days, I guess, but I'm not going to let it bother me."

I was very conscious of the time. I did not want to rush her, but I did want to get to her apartment so we could continue our visit; I guess I let what she said slide right by. When she finished her tea, we drove to her apartment and got settled for our visit. I began to ask her about how she was getting along in it. She replied, but reverted the conversation to her new grandchild, and the fact that her son had not told her. She seemed to look much older as she sat there going over various incidents involving her relationship with her family.

At first I felt annoyed with her for changing the subject and with myself for not redirecting her to the topic. I noticed that as she talked, her eyes were downcast and were often filled with tears. At times she commented half defiantly that she was not going to let things like this bother her, but her nonverbal behaviors indicated the opposite. I was receiving her real message — that of a lonely old lady who was being excluded from the events and activities of her family.

My own goal seemed a bit easier to give up, once I began to be aware of her need to talk about what was on her mind. In another sense, I do not feel particularly comfortable about dumping my plans, because I like to plan and think about my approach with my patients and families. I guess I am saying that I am not the flexible person I thought I was. *That* was the message I got about me. I guess I will have to loosen up a bit, but it does not sound like a very safe, secure role. At any rate, I was glad I was not insistent with Mrs. B., because she really had more important things on her mind. I do not know if listening helped, but it seemed to be what she needed at the time. Next time I visit, I am going to see if she refers to it again before I check it out. Am I getting on the right track?

The nurse in this example clearly had difficulty recognizing the importance of what Mrs. B. was saying and its precedence over the preplanned goal. The nurse's objectives were no less legitimate, however, because many adjustment problems are connected with moving, especially with the elderly. In this incident, however, a priority of need originated from the patient. Such immediate cues should not be overlooked, because the expression of them is based on each person's accumulation of experiences and attitudes. To the extent that each of us experiences a variety of events and feelings, the way we express ourselves — even daily — changes. The subtleties of these behavioral differences are the aspects of communication to which we should be sensitive.

We must learn to "bend with the cue." Old cues and old themes are a part of yesterday. They are generally difficult to recapture, recycle, or reuse for today's interactions (unless the themes are recurrent) and still be pertinent. Flexibility helps us serve a patient's needs *now,* when the immediacy is most strongly felt and most evident. We have the greatest effectiveness when we can "bend" our communication in such a way that our patients *know* we have heard them.

SUMMARY

Whatever communication we implement with our patients, our aim is for it to be both helpful and effective. Specific techniques certainly assist us in our endeavor. They, as all other skills, must be gauged against broader criteria that measure the overall effect of our words and messages upon patients. However eloquent and planned a question or a statement may be, it may prove to be too wordy, too complex, too contradictory, and too rigid in execution. As a result, we receive unrewarding feedback from the patient.

The criteria of efficiency, appropriateness, and flexibility offer us a standard against which to test the effectiveness of our communication. This process is continual and can be used both before and after our contacts with patients. It helps us see how we are progressing and where we need to improve. Like the sequence of events in the therapeutic communication model, all the criteria are engaged in almost simultaneous action and interaction. Thus if we begin by examining our message codes for efficiency, our message content for appropriateness, and our message treatment for flexibility, we have initiated steps to becoming more effective in our communication. The positive feedback we receive from our patients is the validation for those efforts.

NOTES

1. Keltner, John. *Interpersonal Speech-Communication: Elements and Structures,* p. 77.
2. Davis, Anne J. The Skills of Communication, 63:66, 1963.
3. Barnett, Lincoln. *The Treasure of Our Tongue,* pp. 293–294.
4. Barrett-Lennard, G. T. Significant Aspects of a Helping Relationship, 47:227, 1963.
5. Bartlett, John. *Familiar Quotations,* p. 57.

BIBLIOGRAPHY

Barnett, Lincoln. *The Treasure of our Tongue.* New York: Knopf, 1969.
Barrett-Lennard, G. T. Significant Aspects of a Helping Relationship. *Mental Hygiene,* 47:223, 1963.
Bartlett, John. *Familiar Quotations,* 13th ed. Boston: Little, Brown, 1955.
Berlo, David. *The Process of Communication.* New York: Holt, Rinehart and Winston, 1961.
Condon, John C., Jr. *Semantics and Communication.* New York: Macmillan, 1966.
Davis, Anne J. The Skills of Communication. *American Journal of Nursing,* 63:66, 1963.
Keltner, John. *Interpersonal Speech-Communication: Elements and Structures.* Belmont, Calif.: Wadsworth, 1970.
Rogers, Carl R. *Freedom to Learn.* Columbus, Ohio: Merrill, 1969.
Ruesch, Jurgen. *Therapeutic Communication.* New York: Norton, 1961.

V

Channels of Communication

10

Observations

TWO PEOPLE with something to say. Two people inaccessible to each other unless there is some means of transmitting their information. Our sensory and motor skills are the channels that facilitate interpersonal communication, a process that involves the circulation of information both *within* each person (i.e., encoding skills) and *between* people (i.e., encoding and decoding skills). During these exchanges each person monitors his thoughts and transmits them through motor and sensory channels while absorbing and monitoring the messages he receives. As this process takes place, we become increasingly better able to "level, sharpen, and assimilate . . . [message] content in a personally meaningful way" [1]. As a result, interpersonal relationships develop and are strengthened.

Sensory and motor skills are not used separately; each is used in conjunction with others in the simultaneous processes of encoding and decoding during a communication exchange. Thus, observing, listening, touching, and talking are stimultaneous encoding and decoding processes, which we must monitor "to produce the words and gestures [we] intend, [while monitoring] the reactions of others to those words and gestures to see if [our] message prompted the reaction [we] sought" [2].

Channel networks may be multidirectional in that they extend to many other people at once, but here we are concerned primarily with the single channel that permits information to flow between two people — nurse and patient. We have already discussed motor skills, namely, verbal communication, with respect to the nurse as the source-encoder. We still must explore the sensory skills involved in the decoding functions of both nurse and patient, which influence the reciprocal flow of their communication and determine the course of their relationship.

THE ROLE OF OBSERVATIONS

Seeing is believing, or so the saying goes. Seeing is not believing, however, because observation has an inherent selectivity based on our experiences, our senses, and our present frames of reference. What we see therefore, is only a small portion of what is actually taking place; the rest is what we think we see — our internal experience or our interpretation of it. Since each of us has different experiences and interests, our ability to see also differs, even when we are all looking at the same thing. We, therefore, must be taught to see, and in a way that best tells us what is actually taking place as we interact with a patient.

An observation is a factual report of something in our physical world conveyed through one or more of our senses. We then translate the information into thoughts and ideas so that they can be stored for future use. Because observations are a part of our physical reality, we know them to be true in the sense that they exist.

In nursing, accurate description of what we observe is basic to care of the patient. For us, he is the most important person in the physical reality of our professional world. Purposeful observation is necessary to learn what happens to him, what he does, and how he moves and looks. Our observations must be based on what is actually occurring — not what we think or feel has occurred — as detected through our senses. As the description of observable events becomes more accurate, the care given a patient becomes more precise and better suited to his needs.

Observation has several functions in nursing care. It has a supplemental role when it is used with other skills to elicit additional information and description from patients. Observations also function independently as the primary source of data when patients are unable or unwilling to give us the information we need from them. This is the best tactic to use with patients whose behavior is so habitual that they do not notice it, because they would have difficulty sharing something of which they are unaware. Patients who are physically unable to respond verbally make observations of vital importance in gathering data. Similarly, patients may be unwilling to respond verbally in an interview because they feel the questions are too personal or too threatening to them. At these times we may elicit information filled with distortion or exaggeration if we press for answers. Since such information has little value in the formulation of our nursing care, interviewing may have understandable limitations at these times. Finally, observation has a facilitating role, because it is the initial step in the process of problem-solving necessary to the formulation of nursing care based on needs and cues expressed in our presence.

THE DISADVANTAGES OF OBSERVATIONS

Though accurate observations are desirable, there are some drawbacks when they are used in connection with the care of patients. Any activity that is done well takes time, and making observations is no exception. Unlike a straightforward interview, however, which can cover a span of time from the past to the present and into the future, observations can take place only in the present. They can be made only while we are with a patient or participating in an event that includes him. What *has* occurred may have a bearing on him and his care, but that information must be obtained through other methods of data collection, namely, the interview.

Realistically, it is not possible to observe every patient's actions. This forces us to rely on the observations of others (i.e., our co-workers) as they relate to him. We use their comments as an indirect source of information in the planning of nursing care, but we must carefully weigh those comments with respect to attitudinal influences. This introduces elements of error and distortion.

In the problem-solving process, observable data, both physical and emotional, are collected over a period of time to see the kinds of patterns that emerge. From these data, nursing plans are formulated and later implemented. Since time is at a premium in health settings, it is in short supply for deliberative observational tasks. That is not to say that we cannot make accurate observations, but rather our ability to be accurate is severely jeopardized because of the often hurried (and sometimes careless) manner in which we observe our patients.

There is a temptation to generalize from a single observation in our nursing care. What we see once may be atypical or uncharacteristic of the patient's illness or behavior, and if it is used as a basis for action, the resultant care will be unwarranted and inappropriate. Consider the following illustration:

> Mr. W., aged 59, entered the Veterans Administration Hospital for diagnosis of a gastric disorder, which had resulted in a twenty-pound weight loss. He was admitted to a ten-bed ward where patients were ambulatory and responsible for some of their care. The ward was plain and although there were curtains on the windows, there were no curtains or screens around the beds to afford privacy for the patients. The ward was bustling with activity, and the patients were congenial and talkative. Mr. W., on the other hand, was a bachelor who had lived alone in a hotel room for twenty-two years. He was a quiet person who spoke only when approached and then was to the point. Although he did not initiate conversation, he was alert and nonverbally involved with ward activities. The only thing he found difficult was to eat as much as his doctor wished.
>
> The morning of his third day in the hospital, one of the nurses expressed her concern about finding him lying on his bed, facing the wall in an *in utero* position. She also observed that he did not mix well with the other men. Because of these two observations, the nurse called the intern, who read the nurse's notes and wrote a short statement in the progress report

offering a preliminary psychiatric diagnosis because the patient "acts funny." He also ordered a psychiatric consultation.

If the nurse in this example had taken the time to investigate the patient's behavior further, she might not have been so impulsive in reaching her conclusion. In reality, the patient's manner of living was solitary. When he was thrust into a situation in which maintaining privacy was almost impossible, his one recourse was to achieve it by turning his back to others in the ward. Whether or not he was resting or thinking, he was indicating his preference to be left alone for a while, and his intent was honored by the other patients. The conclusions formed by the nurse in this example therefore were inaccurate and invalid. Later the psychiatric consultation corroborated this.

Another drawback of observations is that what we see is filtered through our personal frame of reference. Because of this, our observations are partial and highly selective; we see what suits us at the moment. Most of us engage in such selectivity harmlessly in our everyday activities, but it can be a problem in our interactions with patients. It can assume various forms in our professional work — the patient's light we chose not to see or the patient's discomfort, which does not appear to be too severe. All attest to our limited ability to observe fully and impartially.

The origin of selective observations may be our inability to separate fact from inference. A fact is an event that we witness or experience — something that actually occurs. An inference, on the other hand, is a conclusion drawn from an event or chain of events, which may or may not be related, seen, or experienced. Inferences are not necessarily untrue; they merely indicate a higher or lower degree of probability to the truth. The more widely an inference is shared among us, the greater the probability that it is valid. Remember, this does not mean it is a fact, only that increasing evidence allows us to treat it as if it were a fact. Something that is less predictable is less likely to be valid. Although we may disagree with facts, because of the differences in how each of us experiences the world, what "we get into trouble about are disagreements about inferences which we have stated as if they were facts" [3]. The following brings out the point:

Several sophomore nursing students were allowed to observe a nurse giving an injection into the lower part of a patient's abdomen. The patient was asked to hold her gown up so that the injection would be clearly visible. In doing so, her hands were in view. They were dry and gnarled, making it difficult for her to manipulate her gown. After the injection, the students were asked what they had observed about the patient's hands. One student said she did not notice them because she was watching the injection closely. One student replied, "The woman obviously has arthritis"; another thought that she had been injured.

Here we can see that the fact was that the patient's hands were dry and gnarled. There was agreement about this (except for the nursing student who did not notice), because everyone saw the patient's hands. The notions that she had arthritis or had sustained an injury are inferences and therefore debatable.

All the nursing students witnessed the same event, but they were selective in what they saw and in their interpretation of it. One inference may be right or at least have a higher degree of probability than another, which allows us to act on it as a fact. The students' observations were also partial in that they included only the area around the injection site. Their observations might have been more valid if they had included more of the patient: then they could have relied on what they saw rather than on inferences from the little they did see.

Making observations without relevant knowledge is like seeing our patients through dark glasses. Everyone and everything seems the same, and although we can see shapes and movements, we cannot discern details and colors. Without knowledge, we see without understanding all the subtleties and nuances of each patient with whom we interact. The use of observation implies skill in knowing what to look for and the relationship and significance it has to the patient, his family, and his community. Without such knowledge, our observations, irrespective of our intent, fail in purposeful application.

Lack of visible grief in a mother of another culture may shock our sensibilities, and therefore may be significant *to us,* but the most important thing that should emerge from the observation is that such behavior is socially approved and expected in her culture. This, of course, necessitates knowledge of the family unit in various cultures and the general cultural beliefs, values, and traditions associated with the death of family members.

Knowledge of physical, natural, and social sciences, plus sensory skills, contributes to better perception and description of an individual. Our encoding skills must also be put to use as we sort the unimportant from the significant observations and relay them in a way that describes our understanding of what we have observed. Each interaction with patients needs fresh eyes unobstructed by barriers and knowledge that can add clarity to our observations.

THE OBSERVATION OF NONVERBAL BEHAVIOR

Nonverbal behavior has been described as "an elaborate code that is written nowhere, known by none, and understood by all" [4]. Acted out through a variety of physical movements, gestures, stances, and looks, it conveys, with infinite accuracy, meanings that are only partially transmitted through words. Although verbal behavior is a conscious attempt to communicate, in that we determine the words we use, nonverbal behavior is much harder to control consciously. This may account for our tendency to trust nonverbal behavior rather than words. It may also be the reason scientists have difficulty trying to pinpoint standardized meanings for such behavior.

The nonverbal behavior we observe in patients is, in one sense, literal communication. What is conveyed through our patient's movements is what *really is* for him — not what he thinks he is or what we think he is; it is an on-the-spot message conveyed without verbal frills. A patient may communicate with us nonverbally in a variety of ways. We, therefore, must observe not just with our eyes, but with all our senses, so that we can detect the many ways he reinforces or denies the verbal messages he sends.

It is important to remember the necessity for observing nonverbal behavior in relation to where and with whom it is occurring. The meaning derived from such behavior without consideration for the corresponding situation is like a photograph that freezes an action; the meaning is reduced considerably, because the transitions in behavior, which may indicate a change in attitude or communication, are lost. These changes occur as continuously as our bodies respond to the signals they receive; thus, we have no guidelines and no boundaries to indicate where a nonverbal statement begins and ends. We must observe the harmony or disharmony of all the signals (i.e., behaviors) we are given. These, in turn, provide us with additional insights into the ways nonverbal behavior not only complements our patients' verbal behavior, but also often surpasses it in accuracy and eloquence. As we develop these observational insights we are contributing to our ability to decipher the behaviors we see.

LIFE STYLE

By studying the styles of living that people have adopted, either willingly or involuntarily, we gain insight into the various patterns of living in the community. Though a patient in a semiprivate room or in a ward tells us something of himself as he lives for a while with other patients, his home environment provides us with a more complete picture of how he usually lives and adapts to everyday situations. As more of our energy is invested in the prevention of illness within the community, the observations we make about home environments and family interactions assume greater importance.

Our observations of a neighborhood give us clues to its socioeconomic level, safety, age, cultural makeup, and the accessibility of its services to any one family. Likewise, the design of a home and its furnishings communicate additional information. Some of the factors to consider are the general look of the home (e.g., very neat, casual, or disarrayed), its size and suitability for those who live in it, utilization of space for privacy, work, or play, and the reception given a visitor, particularly if he has professional status or authority. This is often an initial observation; one that is helpful in determining the need for and type of approach that would produce interpersonal comfort.

Our initial observations about other peoples' living quarters and our reactions to them are often carefully noted by patients and their families. Our nonverbal behaviors often reveal attitudes that may influence a family adversely. They then may feel it necessary to apologize to us for their home, for example. Doubtless many of us have done so at some time.

Life styles such as communal living or marriage without legal contract between people of mixed races, of the same race, and between homophiles are becoming more common. The adjustment of these people, particularly when they are subjected to open hostility and rejection from people of more traditional styles of living, has become a health consideration of growing importance within our communities. From the observations we make and share with others, we can learn which aspects of a life style are advantageous and which are detrimental to its participants. These observations are an excellent supplement to the information gained from an interview and assure a more complete picture of a family and its life style.

Problems, whether they are related to drug abuse, nutrition, infectious diseases, education, unemployment, illegitimacy, or child abuse, are faced by all families, irrespective of life style. The way a family accommodates to such situations is reflected by their manner of living. The urban poor, for example, reflect a life style often incomprehensible to many of us. Large families on low incomes, the elderly on fixed incomes, families without a breadwinner — all are struggling to find a compromise in their mode of living. It may reflect priorities with which we disagree, and yet which we must recognize as important based on whatever standard is operative. Home visits allow us to observe regularly whether these priorities help or hinder their life style.

Parent—child interactions, the disciplinary philosophy demonstrated by parents, the role of each parent and child within the home, the way children play with each other, and the toys used and shared in their play communicate some of the aspects of a family's life style. For the elderly, often the placement of inanimate objects, such as plants, scrapbooks, collections of china cups, and other knick-knacks are visible memories of the past, kept alive with each dusting or watering. Hobbies, crafts, and the placement and use of the television indicate the activities that currently occupy their lives. These observations can serve as starting points for discussion of neutral topics; we thereby establish rapport through recognition of interests that are important to the family or individual. Changes in living arrangements and absence of familiar objects, such as furniture, often signal changes before people speak of them. Consider the following example:

> Mrs. B.'s apartment was small and filled with mementos. Her prized possession was an old spinet piano, which had belonged to her grandmother and which she enjoyed playing. After several months of home visits, the nurse noticed that the piano had been removed since her last visit. The room had been rearranged, and although there was more space now, the living room seemed empty without the piano. The nurse wondered what had caused the removal of the piano.

As tea was being served, the nurse verbalized her observation to Mrs. B. Further discussion revealed that she was considering moving into a room in a downtown hotel because she could no longer afford to pay the rent on her apartment. She had a good offer from an antique dealer and took it because she needed the money. Mrs. B. spoke of having to get used to living a new kind of life, which would be hard on her at first because she could take few of her possessions with her to the hotel.

We also develop a life style in our health settings, which indicates to others how we live in our professional environment. When introduced to that style, a patient must not only adjust to another ecological setting, but also change the manner in which he lives. We can observe the adjustments being made and thereby help a patient make the transition with the least amount of difficulty.

Our adjustment to various life styles also is essential, particularly if various aspects of the patient's mode of living are evident in the hospital. For instance, gypsy families may accompany one of their members to the hospital and stay with him day and night. This is not uncommon among practitioners of communal living. Here, a different culture and a particular life style become evident within the hospital.

To many patients, retention of their life style during illness is extremely important to their physical and emotional well-being. Although this may be disruptive or, at the very least, disconcerting to us, the observations we make can give us insight and assist us in being more flexible in similar encounters in the future. A patient's way of life—how he lives it and copes with it — are revealed to us through our observations of him and it is an important component of nursing practice.

POSTURE AND GAIT

The way we stand and move about is a visible signature, a characteristic by which others identify us. From posture we receive information about an individual's perception of himself and about physical problems or limitations. Diseases and injuries may force him to compromise between his usual posture and that which he assumes during illness, such as a bent over, protective bearing.

Posture suggests a person's self-concept by indicating his emotional status at the time of observation. Postures that are stooped, relaxed, awkward, or always erect and seemingly at attention may provide evidence of how a person expresses himself generally. Observable posture that is relatively constant can be considered a nonverbal behavior against which to compare lapses into other types of body stance.

In the book *Body Language* [5], Julian Fast discusses in detail the variety of meanings he feels can be attached to the way we hold and direct the conduct of our bodies. They convey messages which, though often unconscious and subtle, are nevertheless received and responded to by others. The responses, as he indicates in his book, may be a surprise if the sender is unaware of the message implied by his posture. The smoker, for example, relaxed and poised (particularly his hands) while holding a cigarette, can present an opposite picture when he attempts to quit smoking. Then, he may be restless, and his hands and body may be fidgeting.

The way a person walks is related to his posture, because it is a method by which erect bearing is assumed. In whatever area of nursing we may be, we should take the time to step back and observe the ways patients walk. The methods are probably most varied in the hospital, because here patients can be seen using walkers and crutches, walking for the first time without a cast, and walking several days after surgery.

The gaits of persons in other health settings and in the community often go unnoticed if we are not alert to this aspect of nonverbal behavior. The shuffling, slow gait often seen in the elderly, for example, may signify circulatory problems, accommodation to an old fracture, arthritis, pain, the effect of certain drugs, or depression. Whatever the reason, variations in gait are related to health and should be considered in planning interviews. Such was the case in the following example:

> Three times a week, one of the nurses accompanied Mr. W. and Miss T. to see their psychiatrist. Since their appointments were relatively short and followed each other, the nurse waited with them in the lounge, where the doctor's office was located. Each time the psychiatrist came into the lounge, he greeted each patient. He shook their hands and ushered them into the office several steps ahead of him.
>
> When he made rounds on the ward one day, the nurse commented on how good it must make patients feel for him to receive them so kindly and to meet them rather than to wait in the office for them.
>
> "I'm glad you think so," he said, "but I'm afraid I have other reasons as well. I use that time to see how they greet me, and how they are dressed, but mostly to see how they walk and carry themselves. Just watching Mr. W. walk into my office gives me an inkling to his mood. Sometimes, for instance, he walks in very determined and rapidly. I've learned that this means he is anxious or angry, and that most of our time together may well be spent in verbal sparring.
>
> "With Miss T., who's depressed, I watch to see how slow her gait is and how drooped her posture is; together with her apparel she relays to me how badly she may be feeling that day. If it's a pretty bad day, she will find it very difficult to talk, and so I must make more effort to assist her. On the other hand, the more erect and active she is, the more promise there is for a productive session. So you see, greeting them kindly and sincerely is only one part of what I have in mind."

This example reveals how one interview began in the lounge area. It was a preliminary step, which supplemented the interview, and the observations were validated later through verbal communication. Our ability to assess is dependent on how astute we are in making these preliminary observations.

PHYSICAL APPEARANCE

Another aspect of visual communication from which we can profit is personal appearance, which includes our physical characteristics as well as the manner of dress used to complement or contradict them. Dress has been a matter of individual preference dictated over the years by the fashion in vogue. In recent years, however, there has been less devotion to one style and greater freedom of choice, which affords each of us the opportunity to dress in a manner that, in most cases, separates us from others. Variety includes choices in texture, color, design, and cost, and has been extended to both sexes.

Our clothing is a rich source of information about us. In choosing apparel, cosmetics, perfume, aftershave lotion, and jewelry, we supply reliable indicators about ourselves and our personalities. Wearing apparel serves many functions today, among them "protection, concealment, sexual attraction, group identification, display of status and role, self assertion or self-denial" [6]. Current acceptable standards in color and design, for example, would have been considered unacceptable years ago and would have left a person's taste in clothes open to speculation.

Current styles notwithstanding, a community responds to the manners of dress of its members. Some modes are accepted; others are not. People in specific groups, such as Hell's Angels, hippies, religious orders, armed forces, and some health professions are frequently singled out and responded to on the basis of their dress.

Generalizations are easily drawn from such responses, and from them stereotypes are likely to result. If there is little or no contact with a particular group, these pictures may be false and therefore unfair. For example, a man who has long hair and wears old and patched clothes may be stereotyped a hippie, when, in fact, he has had little if anything to do with the hippie movement.

Dress also can signify authority, social position, financial status, religious persuasion, cultural influence, and self-concept. All are observable and all can be useful sources of information in making assessments. Changes in dress can likewise signify an increase in prestige or a loss of self-esteem. There have been many instances in our own lives in which such changes have communicated our thoughts and feelings, such as during illness, or when we are getting ready for a party or simply too tired or depressed to care how we look. These moments and many others influence our patients and families. Finding an elderly woman at home still in her nightgown at 3 p.m., is a good indicator of how she feels. "I have nothing to get dressed for" or "I'm not going anywhere" is what she is telling us nonverbally about her existence.

Physical characteristics also denote the level of health. Mottled skin, cyanotic lips or nailbeds, bruises and wheezing respirations, are a few that are noticeable. Distinguishing physical characteristics such as birthmarks, prominent facial features, height, weight, and deformities also come under our visual scrutiny. Some characteristics are the target of jokes; some are the object of disgust and fear. Others are overlooked altogether. Every person has observable physical characteristics, even if it is only that his height and weight are within normal limits.

Certain colors make some people look unwell. Yellow and beige, depending on the intensity, can make a person look as though he has, or is recovering from, hepatitis. Black, on the other hand, can make people look paler than they really are. If a person who has poor circulation and tends to have cyanotic coloration wears some shades of blue, he may accentuate the blue cast of his skin.

The manner of dress also may conceal less appealing aspects of one's body, thereby distorting or hiding observable characteristics. Maternity clothes, for example, are designed with this in mind. Drug addicts wear long-sleeved blouses or shirts to cover needle marks; dark glasses not only help their eyes adjust to the sun, but also hide dilated pupils — an indication of recent drug use. People who are unsure of their self-concept, are threatened by their sexual identity, or are overweight may dress for concealment also. Men may wear baggy, pleated slacks and long-sleeved shirts, and women may choose loosely hanging dresses, baggy slacks, and bulky sweaters, or keep their coats on during social gatherings.

One must not conclude that a person is trying to conceal something just because his mode of dress fits one of these descriptions; other information must validate such observations. The person with needle marks on his arm is not necessarily a drug addict. He may have been recently hospitalized and have had several intraveneous feedings or blood tests. Ill-fitting clothes may not be so much a sign of concealment as a sign of poverty.

Our perceptions of ourselves are expressed through our bodies in all aspects of our daily lives. We clothe them and use them to interact with other people. They can attract or repel; they can be concealed or distorted, protective or defiant. Whatever they are is a visual form of communication. To the practiced eye the body communicates much, but we must first learn to look and really understand what is being conveyed through its appearance and use.

BUILDINGS AND SETTINGS

Within each community are buildings and settings that influence our interactions with others. Whether or not settings such as parks, vacant lots, and gardens are old or new, they manipulate, in a sense, the type of activity and communication that take place there. Likewise buildings such as churches, schools, and hospitals determine the communication that occurs within them. In other words, they are "areas which individuals enter and in which they behave in accordance with forces that produce the characteristic behavior patterns" [7]. In general, a library is conducive to studiousness and silence, whereas a football game stimulates shouting and cheering. A church may induce a prayerful, thoughtful attitude, whereas a police station might provoke a cautious or antagonistic response. These kinds of expected behavior are consistent, and they give us all a shared frame of reference in our communication.

Architects and city planners are becoming increasingly aware of the significance of walks, gardens, and balconies in the promotion of interpersonal communication (see Figure 16, part G). Miniparks in crowded urban neighborhoods invite interpersonal exchange among children and enable them to have a greater range of healthy life experiences. Unfortunately, we need additional insight into the further effects of buildings and settings have upon us. We have general ideas, however, which can serve as a base for assessing the behaviors that occur in them.

The hospital has long been associated with specific types of conduct. To the patient goes the expected behaviors of helplessness, passivity, and relinquishment of responsibility, in the sense that the only thing he needs to concern himself with is getting well. For us, expected professional conduct includes industry, activity, and responsibility, in the sense that we nurture and care for our patients. In addition, many other types of behavior that do not fall within this category are exhibited in this setting. Actions that contradict our expectations and that indicate our willingness to be passive or lax toward responsibility are observed and imply that we have differing perceptions regarding expected patient behaviors. These behaviors often precipitate open conflict during efforts to communicate.

The hospital, as a symbol of communication, is undergoing change from its traditional image. The patient, as a consumer, assumes a more active role as he becomes more aware of his right to health care and information. We are beginning to see new health settings develop within the community, where unexpected or atypical behavior is the norm. There, the conventional views of role, status, and authority are being altered. Interpersonal communication is encouraged and, in a good many instances, sought out by health professionals. This is the setting where one can observe the various types of behaviors that are typical of and expected in that neighborhood.

Buildings such as hospitals, on the other hand, are what we make them, and in some of them, activity that would promote interpersonal sharing is discouraged. In some, patients are prohibited from visiting between wards; in others, very little space is available for a solarium. Beyond watching television or reading, many patients have no space for recreation. These architectual oversights (some of which are based on financial considerations) can and do influence interpersonal communication among patients.

The changes that take place in these settings are in part due to the visibility of interpersonal behaviors. Such observations enable us to learn how people interact and how those interactions can be improved.

FACIAL EXPRESSIONS

No body part is more expressive than the face. Each muscle is primed to help form an expression, of which there are endless possibilities. The face captures attention because it supplies obvious and subtle cues, which assist us in decoding the messages we receive through other channels. The facial accompaniment to a verbal message, for example, can either reinforce the information or refute it. The face, as an instrument of expression, is also elusive because of the variety of moods and feelings it can convey.

Whatever the expression, one facial cue should not be the only source of information. The more cues we observe, whether postural or environmental, the more valid our conclusions. Two factors to consider in the observation of facial expressions are the setting in which the cue is communicated and its context among other faces. A person who is smiling tells us very little, because the meaning could range from contentment to sardonic amusement. In the setting of a party, however, among people who are visibly enjoying themselves, the person who is smiling conveys something more specific. On the other hand, if the faces of other people do not indicate enjoyment, we may draw other conclusions.

Eye contact is also a vital part of one's facial expression. When we observe others, we too are observed, and in this way, basic and mutual understanding develops. Visual contact among people often prefaces a message. In glancing at others, we inform them of our involvement or willingness to communicate, of the absence of suspicion, and of our fear or hostility. In averting someone's eyes, we indicate our unwillingness to initiate or maintain social contact or our withdrawal from the suggestions, arguments, commands, intimidations, or affection of others [8]. Dominance can also be communicated through mutual glances, depending on how long one person can maintain eye contact with another. The person who looks away first has, in a sense, given in, thereby indicating the dominance of the other person. It is also asserted when the eyes are not on an equal level, as in the case of a nurse who is standing and looking down at a bedridden patient.

Eye contact in a relationship can be significant in preserving one's ego. For example, one usually avoids another's eyes when asked very personal or embarrassing questions. By signaling a lessening of involvement in the relationship, we reduce "the intensity of shame, guilt or fear experienced during threatening interpersonal exchanges" [9]. Such threats also are noted when people are too close. More physical distance is created by not meeting the other person's eyes. As spatial distance increases, visual contact is restored in an effort to reduce interpersonal distance.

Mutual eye contact is visual conversation, the message and context of which are continually being modified. Our close interactions with patients enable us to see the many ways they use their eyes for communication and to discover that their messages often are significant. Whatever the specific information exchanged through eye contact, it generally serves to "signal information-seeking, indicate that the channel is open, permits concealment or exhibitionism, shows recognition of social relationships and reflects approach-avoidance motivation" [10].

Facial expressions, including the use of our eyes, significantly contribute to our understanding of the subtleties and complexities of nonverbal behavior. No one expression can be categorized accurately unless we take into account accompanying physical cues that reinforce it. The message we receive via another's facial expression subsequently affects the way we begin, maintain, and conclude our communication with him.

Although conscious control of all our facial expressions is impossible, we can try to become more aware of those that affect the communication of our patients. Just as we may have to exercise flexibility in altering our communication approach in response to a patient's facial cues, we should also try to respond to whatever he may be indicating about our facial expressions. This feedback can help us determine our success in trying to be congruent in our communication.

HANDS AND GESTURES

Our hands are another expressive part of our bodies. Like our faces, the musculature of our hands provides us with a great variety of movements, which are too numerous to be cataloged accurately. The ways hands are used and the messages conveyed with them vary with the culture and the environment. Americans, for example, tend to use hands and gestures for purposes of activity, whereas, among Italians, it serves as illustration, and among the French, it expresses style and containment [11].

In gesturing, our hands become visual italics, emphasizing, punctuating, and clarifying our verbal communication. Alone, they indicate feelings, attitudes, and ideas that are not being expressed verbally. Wringing the hands and pronounced mannerisms involving them, for example, may indicate anxiety; hand movements used by mimes, such as Marcel Marceau, can create impressions of people experiencing a variety of emotions.

Gestures are a great asset to our interpersonal exchanges, but they also have negative aspects. For example, they can convey messages that are detrimental to the development of healthy interpersonal relationships. The substitution of manual expression for verbal expression (except in instances of physical limitations) may indicate a person's withdrawal from interpersonal involvement and a regression to more primitive patterns of behavior.

Miss C., aged 30, had been confined to the state hospital for the past five years. She was extremely withdrawn and for the most part was mute. When she did communicate, her verbal responses were monosyllabic. Over the years, though still withdrawn and quiet, she began to be more active. Her communication with the staff at this time was conducted in silence. Whenever she wanted something, Miss C. gestured and received what she wanted from the staff, who by this time had decoded her hand signals. For example, when Miss C. wanted a cigarette, she held up her right forefinger and middle finger, and promptly received her cigarette. This method of communication was continued by the aides who manned the nursing stations despite the fact that Miss C. could and did verbally communicate and was seen doing so to her parents over the phone.

Although the expressiveness of our hands, whether in gesture or activity, usually corresponds to the current task or conversation, not all gesticulation is used appropriately. In some forms of mental illness, for example, gestures signal a disturbing conflict, which is often unconscious. Two reasons for this may be that they lack an external referent (that is, they are not connected to any specific concrete act) and they do not appear to serve any immediate adaptive goal [12].

The ways we use our hands for activity or for gestures are not standardized. Although there is universality in certain body activities, such as sitting and standing, no two people do so in the same way. Likewise, while the motions we use to emphasize and clarify our verbal communication may reinforce what we say, one gesture has a different significance for each person using it. Our observations of patients, therefore, must encompass the unique expression of each gesture in conjunction with his pattern of communication.

SLEEP

Among the many activities in which man participates, the one least understood is sleep. Despite the climate, culture, or time, the ritual of sleep is universally experienced by all people. Embedded in this ritual are scientific data, which have only begun to be explored by health professionals. Initial studies have shown, among other things, that: sleep is not a state of oblivion or unconsciousness, but a sequence of rhythmic cycles, each having different phases with specific neutral functions; *all* people dream at periodic intervals every night and must do so in order to maintain a delicate physiological and psychological balance, as yet not fully understood; sleep is punctuated by a series of rapid eye movements (called REM sleep) as well as other similar activity, which is detectable on measuring devices, such as electroencephalographs, electrocardiographs, myographs, and thermometers. The many questions arising from the preliminary research need to be explored and studied to unravel the mysteries of sleep.

Sleep, as a much-needed restorative process for patients, is often overlooked or underestimated in our attempts to systematically collect data through observations. At best, our perceptions of a patient engaged in sleep are cursory and assumptive. If he has his eyes closed and is lying quietly, we conclude that what we see is good, in the sense that he is enjoying a night of sound sleep. Yet, we are often contradicted by his own assessment that his night's sleep may have been less than satisfactory.

Two decades ago we had little specific information about sleep habits upon which to base our observations. With the discovery that sleep occurs in a series of cycles, each lasting from 90 to 120 minutes and each having its own set of patterns, our observations can now be aligned to the systematic approach involved in the problem-solving process. Although we cannot easily detect the many precise changes that occur during a patient's sleep cycle (scientific instruments can do this), we can observe the sleep patterns methodically at the gross level. Physiological changes are observable during intervals of stillness, and include muscle twitches, eye movements, facial expressions, body and respiratory movements.

Recent information gleaned from preliminary research has indicated a relationship between certain illnesses and a patient's sleep pattern.

> [This information] may exert a powerful influence on our behavior, attention shifts, ability to work, response to illness, even our capacity to survive. Hospital personnel, for instance, make the casual observation that the predawn hours are often the fatal ones for critically ill people. They are a time of many coronaries . . . If indeed, most patients are highly vulnerable during the dawn and early morning hours, some changes in hospital schedules might be warranted . . . [a group of physicians] suggested that surgery should not be scheduled too early in the morning if possible and that the traditional hospital regimen may disturb patients too early [13].

Various medications may significantly alter the sleep patterns of our patients, thereby affecting the quality of their rest. For example, sedation often produces less restful sleep than we realize. A patient's inability to sleep may have metabolic or neural origins, requiring sleep medications to be prescribed with greater selectivity so that they induce and maintain sleep during the night with minimal alterations in the various stages [14]. Several barbiturates, for example, suppress the initial stage of sleep (i.e., Stage I-REM). Depending on the illness, the suppressive tendency of these barbiturates can potentiate other hazards to the patient's physical well-being.

Prescribing medications for sleep has little value if it is not followed up by observation of its effects on patients. This task will become increasingly important as the relationship between drugs and sleep becomes clearer. In the meantime, we must continue to do whatever we can to ensure that a patient's sleep is achieved. This may necessitate efforts to curtail noises, which are prevalent at night, and in which we play no small part. The primary area of focus, however, will continue to be interpersonal communication, for it is here that we can initiate nursing actions to promote rest and sleep without resorting to medication. Unexpressed anxiety, lack of ventilation, and physical discomfort are just a few of the factors that interrupt the cyclic progress of a patient's sleep. The more we learn about the activity and its effect upon people, the more we will be able to observe intelligently the sleep patterns of our patients and to implement appropriate nursing measures when needed.

THE TEST OF OBSERVATIONS

There is great satisfaction in knowing that some object, event, or person really exists. Our security and our confidence in ourselves and in the world increase as we become more sure of their dependability. Knowing the existence of an object, event, or person is not magical; it is achieved through inquiry, by which our initial premise is confirmed or refuted. This procedure is called verification, and we must use it to substantiate the validity of our observations of patients.

One of the basic errors we make in observing patients is in assuming that what we see is true. From such assumptions we make inferences (i.e., we draw conclusions) upon which we base our nursing care. Assumptions are statements we make about reality that are unproved and questionable. Drawing conclusions from such dubious evidence is a sign of faulty reasoning, the product of which can only be nursing care of questionable value.

Earlier we defined an observation as a fact that has a direct, visible relationship to the physical world. It is this initial step that must be verified; then inferences may follow in two ways: one, by gathering together verified facts about a problem and from them drawing a general conclusion that explains them (this is called inductive reasoning), or two, by proceeding from a general premise that has been proved and drawing specific conclusions based on that premise (this is called deductive reasoning). In both types of inferences, as we can see from the definition, verification is the first step in the chain of events that proceeds from the identification of the nursing problem to the solution. Let us consider some of the means by which we can test the validity of our observations.

We said earlier that although observations have independent functions, they best serve as supplemental data for interviews, because in the exchange of information we learn the validity of our observations. With time and continued sharing, patterns can emerge that further substantiate our observations and lend more credibility to the inferences we may make.

Inquiry through the use of various communication skills helps elicit verbal and nonverbal agreement, depending on our approach. A closed question, for example, may be responded to verbally or nonverbally, such as in "Did you drop this book?" Similarly, by verbally labeling what we have seen, we not only elicit more verbal information from a patient, but also provide him with a source of recognition and of concern. Comments that include sensory verbs facilitate verification, such as: "I noticed that you hadn't eaten very much today"; "You look tired"; "I see you're limping more than usual."

Prefacing our questions with a brief description of what we have observed establishes a frame of reference for a patient and gives him a better idea of how to respond. For example, "I noticed you wiping your eyes and blowing your nose a few minutes after visiting hours. You also looked a little sad. What has happened?"

Verification of our observations, by whatever communication skills we employ, is done in the interest of achieving accuracy. Any method we use to collect information, however, is apt to be imprecise, and accuracy may not be totally realized because of the time and effort required. We then must select a method of data collection that will give us the greatest precision within our limits of time. Observations, therefore, may not be useful if they are the primary source of data. Accuracy in observation comes through the practice of refining them within a time span that will be economic to our efforts and ultimately benefit our patients.

NOTES

1. Barnlund, Dean. Interpersonal Communication: Survey and Studies, p. 245.
2. Ibid., p. 230.
3. Kaiser Aluminum News. *Communications*, p. 30.
4. Barnlund, op. cit. (note 1), p. 536.
5. Fast, Julian. *Body Language.*
6. Barnlund, op. cit. (note 1), p. 518.
7. Ibid., p. 512.
8. Ibid., p. 534.
9. Ibid., p. 535.
10. Ibid., p. 535.
11. Ibid., p. 531.
12. Ibid., p. 532.
13. U.S. Department of Health, Education and Welfare. *Current Research on Sleep and Dreams*, p. 6.
14. Foss, Grace. Sleep, Drugs and Dreams, p. 2319.

(Bibliography appears at end of Chapter 13.)

Listening

LISTEN TO THE SOUND of words and the noises, which are all about us. Auditory symbols fill our ears; they are stimuli that need to be sorted and understood, and to which we must respond. Sounds full of meaning, yet often disguised by words and motives hiding subjects too painful, too revealing, or too difficult to share directly. Listen to them — they come from our patients.

They tell us about themselves in a way that *never* says exactly what they mean, and yet *always* conveys what they mean. When we listen to our patients we do so consciously, voluntarily entering into a world of thought and feeling many times foreign from our own, but that we must learn to understand. It is a world that daily bombards us with a variety of aural as well as other sensory stimuli, all of which must be perceived and sorted so that we can respond with comprehension and meaning. This dynamic process of attaching significance to what we hear is called listening. Of all the skills we practice in relating to our patients, it is the primary sensory skill we use to effect therapeutic communication with them.

Listening is a highly specialized perceptual process in which we learn to select stimuli (usually auditory and visual) in our interactions that are useful in guiding an interview and, in turn, the patient's care. Generally, we exercise selectivity throughout our lives, because it is simply impossible to absorb all the stimuli we perceive. In our interactions, the sphere of our attention and interest is limited to the environment of the patient because of his need or illness, and we focus on consciously selecting the information related to it.

By focusing our attention within this sphere, we are immersed in the patient's frame of reference, totally concentrating on it so that we may understand how he perceives the world. We must, in a sense, put on his spectacles so that we can view reality in the same way [1]. To do this, we must set aside our own spectacles and, for the time we are needed, temporarily relinquish our ideas, our perceptions, and our world.

As we assume another frame of reference — as we relinquish our ideas and our perceptions — we begin to learn what is important to him and how he conveys it through the aural symbols of words and sounds. We begin to learn how he uses words to evade, to disguise, and to express pleasure and affection, just as we learn to listen for the meaning of what he does not say or is unable to say.

We must have willingness and purpose, for these factors have great significance in determining not only our own listening behavior, but also the extent to which a patient shares himself with us. Both factors suggest a commitment to the application of selectivity, i.e., carefully choosing information from a patient that will help us to understand him and his needs. These, in turn, are the basis for the quality of nursing care he will receive, assuming that we have some idea or goal upon which to focus.

It is not easy to immerse ourselves in what a patient is saying, because we initially choose to listen to the things that we wish to hear or that we feel are important, regardless of what other, perhaps more significant, things he may be saying. For these reasons, in our beginning efforts to listen, we think that to do so effectively is an extraordinarily simple task, and we are puzzled by the emphasis that is placed upon it in nursing.

THE FACTORS IN LISTENING

Listening is not a static process. It fluctuates constantly, scanning the infor-mation we absorb and retaining, even on an unconscious level, almost everything that reaches our ears. The information we do not use today we store for future use when we want to help our patients recreate past experiences. What does it take to mentally transport ourselves and our imagination into a patient's percep-tion of the world? Though we absorb much through listening, the conscious selectivity required to make our attempts more beneficial is dependent on a variety of factors.

Being attentive to what a patient may be saying does not imply interest. The two should be synonymous, but they are not. Interest implies that we are other person oriented; we are concerned with his needs, problems, and expectations. These purposes are exemplified in all aspects of therapeutic communication, not the least of which is listening. The interest, and with that, the corresponding attention we give each patient, sets the tone of the verbal communication he shares with us in the future.

Though each patient may have inherent or intuitive criteria for determining how interested another person is in him, those standards are based on nonverbal behaviors. The way we sit or stand, our ability to maintain attentive eye contact, the way we nonverbally acknowledge what he says, and the level of our distractibility all indicate our sincerity of purpose and level of interest. Because such behaviors are deliberately (in the sense of purposefully) used during interaction with a patient, it is relatively easy for him to determine just how interested we are. That is the reason we need to become oriented to other people. Again, our ability to focus attention and interest on our patient bears great significance to what he shares with us and the way he does it.

Since the listening process implies interpersonal exchange, it is also a process that requires participation. The degree of participation coincides with the level of interest, because it demonstrates our willingness to enter into a realm of experience outside ourselves. The role of a participatory listener is one in which we sincerely engage ourselves with another person. In that sense, we must listen not only to him, but also to ourselves, because we cannot really respond to another person unless we are listening to him.

Taking part in the activity of listening also requires time for that participation to mature into mutual respect and understanding. An expenditure of time is required for participation to become a nursing activity of substance. We therefore must have a sense of purpose in each moment we spend with a patient, because time is at a premium.

Listening, as a nursing activity, often is on the lower end of an interpersonal hierarchy of skills. Although it has received major emphasis in the understanding and development of helping relationships, in nursing practice it often is supplanted by more immediate and visually apparent tasks or priorities. Listening skillfully during a nursing task is often a good utilization of time, but as a solitary activity (except perhaps with psychiatric patients) it is often considered unessential. Activity is connected with movement, and physical movement means doing things. Anything that cannot be seen via movement is readily confused with nonactivity. Listening is an activity we equate with time and movement — two items of importance in nursing practice. Conscious selectivity within the listening process by its definition necessitates time as a temporal dimension and as an expenditure.

Time means availability, in the sense that we indicate willingness to our time for the patient's benefit. In a milieu of rushing about, urgent tasks, and endless demands for our time, energy, and skills, our availability for the purpose of listening has considerable impact on patients. An unwilling offer of time predetermines the course of our communication and is inconsistent with our professional aims.

Beyond showing interest in our patients, participating with them, and willingly listening to them, the information we seek must have meaning for us if it is to have any effect in our nursing practice. That meaning comes from an under-standing of our patients' communication, which we achieve by developing and testing theories of human behavior, with consideration for the various physiological and psychological processes involved.

Just as practice is necessary to become skillful in listening, it cannot exist without knowledge so that we can compare what we have absorbed. The attachment of meaning, which makes listening an act separate from hearing, is possible only when we have knowledge upon which to base it. If we are unable to perceive a patient's need and relate it to nursing theory, he will have shared his thoughts and perceptions without purpose. To ensure against this, we must exercise all our personal and professional responsibility to see that the focus of our attention is not wasted effort.

One element can easily be overlooked in the listening process, and that is risk. Each time we enter into another person's frame of reference, put on his spectacles, and see the world through his eyes, we surrender not only our world but also a part of ourselves to another's thoughts and feelings. When this occurs, we run the risk of being changed by the experiences we are encountering.

If the listening process has any meaning for us during interactions with patients, we must become aware that it is a period of time during which we must suspend judgment and resist the temptation to evaluate on the basis of it.

Putting on another's spectacles, even temporarily, helps us better understand points of view different from our own. In doing so, however, we become vulnerable in the sense that we relinquish our protected selves, and leave ourselves open to another. Such exposure introduces us to the possibility of being changed by the situation we have entered. In an age in which change is a predictable and often accelerated element of our society, we have learned to organize and protect ourselves with values, attitudes, and beliefs, which anchor us firmly within secure boundaries. Courage and a sense of personal calm and security are required to extend ourselves beyond the familiar and into an interpersonal unknown. Each attempt, no matter how brief, changes us — alters our perceptions of the world and of ourselves.

It is the risk we *must* take, however, when we perceive that, in so doing, we may gain more than we may lose with respect to a patient's trust. The more risks we take and the more we listen to a patient, the more effort he is willing to make in expressing his ideas and perceptions clearly. At these times, it is not uncommon for him to gain greater understanding of his concerns because he has articulated his ideas.

No single factor functions alone in listening effectively to patients; they must all be present and coordinated. When interpersonal communion is established, the influence of listening extends far beyond the ordinary exchanges of everyday encounters and affords us rare glimpses of the understanding that can exist between two people. The following story of a nursing student and an elderly woman serves as an illustration:

What exactly did I listen to? I heard an older woman tell me about a period of grief which she was going through. It was the first anniversary

of the death of a very close friend. She told me the story of their relationship, the details of his death, and her attempts to get over it. During
this time, she gained weight and her blood pressure rose, which did not
make her feel happier.

Now I must attach some meaning to what I heard. I first tried to discover if it was possible the fear of death upset her. From what she said
in response, I ruled this out.

The more I listened to her, the more I found out that she must have
wanted to talk to somebody and tell them about it — somebody uninvolved
in the event. The only other people she could relate it to were people who
were involved and who passed judgment on her. She was tired of keeping
it inside herself and wanted to get it off her chest. I let her know I wanted
to listen — just listen and not pass judgment.

What really impressed me was the fact that she did not force me to
listen. She tactfully dropped hints, which she wanted me to pursue, but
she more or less gave me a choice as to whether I wanted to hear her out.
When I did respond and show interest, she shared her feelings with me.

Although I was primarily the listener, she saw to it that it was not a
one-way conversation. She responded to my words of encouragement
and let me know what I said was important to her, too.

After that visit, I began to see what a skill listening is. What a significant difference there is between hearing and listening. Making her feel
worthy and letting her know that what she was saying was important to
me, and was not going in one ear and out the other, encouraged her to
open up even more. When she knew that I was really willing to give my
time and attention to her problem, she in turn felt she was not wasting
my time by sharing all her troubles with me for an hour. The more she
opened up, the more relaxed she became.

LISTENING AS ASSESSMENT

Identification of Themes

A helping relationship is made up of daily interactions, each offering us additional fragments of information about a patient. Just as one interaction can
provide us with new insights, a series of exchanges can give shape and substance
to the aspects of a patient's personality that form the common core of his behaviors. These are expressed verbally and nonverbally in a variety of ways, such as
the way a robe is placed and the kinds of books read. All communicate behavior
that has meaning for the person engaged in it and the one observing it.

There is a common core of beliefs, feelings, and ideas in each patient's verbal
communication. It is sometimes blatant, sometimes subtle, but it is always
present. These common cores are called themes — unifying, repetitive thoughts
or motifs that connect the various forms of expression, as in music and poetry.

Feelings and attitudes that are not expressed also have themes. Their absence
indicates significance for a patient. What he does not say or do is often of
greater importance than what he communicates overtly. The way he verbally

expresses himself is also an area needing our attention. The contradictions between his verbal and nonverbal behaviors, tone of voice, pet words or phrases, pitch, pace, and inflection all are important in assessing the significance of a message, and all comprise the feeling tone of a patient's communication.

Whether or not a patient's messages are obvious or subtle, stated or unexpressed, the skill of listening involves us actively in ferreting out unifying cores of behavior. As an assessment task, it is of major importance in this respect.

Though themes are always present in a patient's communication, their significance is often expressed through variations in the basic theme. Themes, therefore, are not always identifiable through overt behaviors. The greater the ego-threat, the greater the need (albeit unconscious) to disguise the impact and perception of the threat in a maze of subtle or symbolic communication. Until the patient has a feeling of interpersonal safety, the variations of his particular theme are a protective means of testing our intentions in developing a helping relationship. New variations may be revealed in each successive interaction; one day the theme may be evident and the next day barely perceptible, yet it persists.

A theme may center on deeply felt problems (either known or unrecognized); it may relay basic perceptions of one's own personality, of one's feelings of self, or of attitudes toward significant others. Words, as one patient remarked, are not always what they seem; they are decorations on a tree to make things prettier and easier. The translation of a deeply felt concern requires words and behavior which disguise feelings through the use of prettier and easier modes of expression.

Because of the infinite variety of ways one theme can be communicated by one patient, we must be actively involved in the listening process, not only through our senses, but also through the encoding and decoding skills we have acquired in nursing practice. These areas within the therapeutic communication model enable us to see relationships in the communications we receive, thereby helping us exercise selectivity.

What is it then that we must begin to discern about the various decorations of a patient's communication? There are many to consider. Tone of voice, the quality of voice through which feeling is expressed, is one revealing aspect of communication. It may sound cheery, sad, abrupt, amusing, clipped, or hesitant, to name a few examples. In addition, tone is the channel through which we detect the incongruency between what a patient says and what he means.

The pacing of one's communication, that is, the rhythm of the words, can indicate the manner in which a patient approaches a subject. The rapidity of speech used by a speaker can, for example, indicate whether it is his usual pattern of speech or a means he uses to activate a listener's interest. An apparent lack of rhythm, such as in monotonous cadences, may suggest a difficulty with emphasis. Sometimes fear or anxiety can precipitate monotonous speech patterns, like those noticed in speaking before a large audience. At other times, a person's intrapsychic problems may deplete energies otherwise used for animated expression. It is often hard to keep our attention focused on what these people are trying to say without betraying ourselves.

The relevance of a patient's verbal communication is another important area for us to consider in developing our listening skills. The messages may not always appear to fit the circumstances, and in this regard, there is a similarity between the criterion we use to measure both our effectiveness and the appropriateness of what a patient shares with us. Various situational or intrapsychic factors may account for the inappropriate lapses in a patient's communication, and they may have dual meanings for the patient as well as for ourselves.

A patient may verbally communicate some message, which in terms of an interpersonal situation may be inappropriate, yet it may express a problem appropriate to his need, but that he cannot deal with directly. We often react to the inappropriate content rather than to the underlying need. A patient's reasons for communicating in this manner may be varied, but often they represent some form of ego-threat that is sufficiently dangerous to require altering the usual manner of communication.

Not all patients are conscious of this process or of the need that has precipitated it. In some situations, this modification may seem playful, innocent, or innocuous, but if it persists, we must intervene upon it. An example of one such occasion follows:

A patient, Mr. J., aged 28, was convalescing from a severe heart attack, his first serious illness. He was a construction worker who was highly regarded by his firm. He had been married for eight months prior to his hospitalization.

About the sixth week of his convalescence, various nursing students began to complain to their instructor and to the head nurse about the suggestive and offensive remarks he was making to them. Since he was in a four-bed ward, his comments were loud enough to be heard by the other patients, who thought they were funny and encouraged him in this behavior. Mr. J. succeeded in embarrassing the students, who were at a loss to stop his remarks. As a result, they became angry with him and did not wish to be assigned to him. The patient's remarks were focused upon the nursing students who were sophomores and juniors; older students and the nursing staff members were not troubled with this behavior.

A nursing conference was held to discuss Mr. J.'s behavior and its effect upon the students. Information received from the doctor revealed that plans for discharge were being discussed and included allowing his return to the construction firm in a different capacity. These discussions between the doctor and Mr. J. seemed to coincide with the behavior the students disliked.

The students' admitted that they felt helpless in dealing with Mr. J., particularly since they considered it their duty. In not being able to meet their own role expectations, they felt threatened and inadequate. Their instructor suggested that Mr. J. might be experiencing the same feelings, and though she realized that her hunch needed validation, it might be the key to understanding his behavior.

The instructor continued, "Here we have a young man with everything to look forward to — a very good job, one that takes a good deal of physical ability, recognition by his peers and his boss, and a young wife to whom he has been married just eight months. Central to all of these things is the factor of his masculinity, that is, his role as a breadwinner and husband. Suddenly he has a severe heart attack at a very early time in his life — too early really. He has what many of us consider an illness of middle age, or an old man's disease. It's an illness you can often expect after you have lived a little and accomplished what you have set out to do."

"I wonder how a 28-year-old man takes it? Does he begin to see himself as an invalid — someone who is over the hill? What does this do to his self-concept and his role expectations? What happens to his job? Will he end up pushing a pencil instead of a hammer? And what about his home life? Will he feel as though he can still be a husband to his wife?"

"These may be the kinds of things he is worrying about, and your presence as young women only reminds him of his loss of role. This may be too painful for him to look at right now. The easiest way might be to assert his idea of masculinity, which seems to be through suggestive comments, stated in the presence of other males, who give him recognition and affirmation as a man, all the while dominating students who, at the same time, are not too sure of their own roles, both professional and personal."

"What we need to consider in our nursing approach is how we can discourage the behavior without rejecting the man. Let's discuss this with his doctor, and tomorrow plan on specific nursing actions through which we can validate and accomplish our nursing goals."

We must listen to the ways a patient misuses words; perhaps he does not speak English well, or he tries to use complicated words or phrases without understanding them. Notice the way a patient uses slang, the repetition of certain words or phrases, such as *me* or *they* in reference to persons involved in some misunderstanding. Repetition can indicate a theme needing further exploration with the patient.

Frequent use of phrases such as, "I wish", "I rely", "I expect", "I desire", or "I hope" may indicate a theme of optimism, which would be important to foster in our interactions with him. Likewise, helplessness and dejection are suggested in phrases such as: "There's no point"; "What's the use?"; "Don't bother"; "Stop fussing"; and "I'm not very good company." The diversity of language used to convey or to suggest a theme is endless; we, therefore, must expect diversity when we listen to our patients.

Familiarity with a patient's ability to use language is a prerequisite to accommodating our verbal communication to his level of understanding and usage. The content patients offer us verbally often is devoid of the niceties of middle-class euphemisms. They often say what they mean in words explicit with description, a good many of which may offend our unaccustomed ears. It may be the language of their culture, their gang, their race, or their profession, and within that framework it is both amusing to them and futile for us to use other, nicer words. For example, a prostitute who comes to a clinic asking for health care because she got the clap from a trick is not referring to any magic act; she is talking about having contracted gonorrhea from one of her clients.

We have many such vocabularies with which we must become knowledgeable, and at times we must use them if we are to be understood and accepted. We are not likely to be as effective if we persist in using words and terms too complicated or too nice to be understood. We must listen for the way a patient uses phrases that are important in a particular health care situation. We will receive only a blank stare if we use the term *void* when the patient uses other words that refer to urination.

We must not take offense at the vernacular, the colorful, or the explicit. If these terms are better understood by our patients because of upbringing, cultural background, or some other factor, we should be prepared to use them. This means, of course, that in the process of listening to many patients, we begin to acquaint ourselves with the unique and colorful vocabularies that are used (and with great effectiveness) by a large segment of people in our communities.

Pertinent to the identification of themes are verbal and nonverbal cues that entice us into further assessment by means of repetition. Key words that a patient may use, often unknowingly, suggest attitudes that pervade his perception and his problem. Phrases such as "no one cares" and "people are no good" suggest an area of perception that may benefit from exploration and description. A patient's words — how he sees his situation and describes it — help us to further assess the importance of the topic under discussion.

In the following example, a nursing student visiting Mrs. C., a 92-year-old lady, suggested additional home visits by one of the nuns from a nearby parish. The nuns had a visiting program and could help Mrs. C. in managing her apartment.

> Mrs. C. immediately changed the topic to a discussion of the awful way in which animals are butchered. She launched into a five-minute tirade against all people who eat meat and don't give "two shakes" about how it is obtained. While listening to Mrs. C.'s condemnation of the meat industry, I was trying to determine why she jumped from the subject of a visiting nun to that of meat.
>
> In my naiveté, I concluded that her mental processes were changing before my eyes, and thus she was not thinking clearly at all. Little did I realize just *how* clearly the dear lady was thinking. Her next comment blew that theory sky high. She said, "The Christians are the worst of them. More atrocities have been committed in the name of Christianity than any other. Christians eat meat right and left with absolutely no

regard for the sinful way in which the poor animals have been killed. I just don't understand Christians, not at all!"

By this time, I realized that Mrs. C. was talking about something very important to her. It seemed that she was afraid that because she didn't understand Christianity, Christians certainly would not understand or accept her since she was an agnostic. A visit by a nun therefore might well be out of the question. I further realized that my response would be of great importance and my words must be well chosen. I said, "Are you trying to tell me that you feel the sisters won't accept you and may try to convert you?"

Her response indicated that I had understood her correctly. She said, "That is exactly right, dear. All you Christians are out to convert the world, with no regard for individual people and their feelings. You presume that all non-Catholics are wrong, and you are going to show them the right way if it is the last thing you do!"

What could I say? I knew that I must tell her that things were changing, but I had to do it in a very understanding way, showing her that I really listened to what she had said. "I'm sure that this is the picture you've received over the years," I said, "but the ideas of Christianity are undergoing tremendous changes. Perhaps in getting acquainted with the sisters, you will be able to see for yourself." She seemed to accept this explanation for the present.

The thematic components of a patient's message are not always communicated verbally, even though the message may be direct. Often the theme is suggested by what is not said — by subjects that are avoided and by the "sounds of silence," which may reveal far more eloquently the patient's feelings and attitudes. These "sounds" may reaffirm his verbal communication, or they may give us a different picture of him.

Nevertheless, the feeling tones, that is, the underlying secondary information transmitted through the feelings the patient may be experiencing at the time, often more accurately express his message. Through such feeling tones, we can discover and verify a number of emotional states, such as anger, fear, happiness, jealousy, pride, sadness, and satisfaction [2]. The list of emotions could be endless, but before discussing them, we must consider the sensitivity we need in order to identify and delineate the feelings at the core of their communication.

Regardless of whether a patient chooses to communicate verbally or nonverbally, directly or indirectly, sparingly or profusely, we must develop listening behaviors that actively support these attempts and demonstrate that during the moments of sharing we are unequivocally with him. We may do this by nodding, uttering sounds of acknowledgement, or establishing attentive eye contact. These behaviors indicate a process of activity — of interpersonal communion, which each patient must feel he can rely on when we are with him.

Listening is assessment — a sensory tool which, when developed and used consistently, helps us attach meaning to a patient's ideas, regardless of how they are communicated. Listening is always a process of discovery — of finding relationships between what is said and what is not conveyed directly. The discovery of meaning through listening means refraining from jumping to conclusions; it means not being content with the label, but realizing the significance of the behavior behind it. It also means patience in sifting a variety of messages and selecting from them the ideas that are important to pursue. Discovery involves awareness of how our perceptions and feelings influence our ability to listen and, at the same time, affect the patient's willingness to continue sharing.

Preoccupied with *nursing* goals that have become integral to nursing education and practice, we sometimes lose sight of our *patient's need* to communicate with a caring, listening, and helping person. Because of the stress of illness and the uncertainty of the future, patients have an overwhelming need to reach out to other human beings, and they try many ways to capture our attention. At these times the important elements in the activity of listening are the availability and sensitivity we extend to patients when they feel the need to talk to someone. The signals we relay to them are visible acknowledgement of that need.

Common Themes

Listening for themes is an important function in the assessment of patients' needs. The number of themes seems endless when consideration is given to the different way any one of them can be communicated. The following themes do not cover the spectrum of possibilities; they merely suggest areas of which we should be aware as we develop our listening skills during encounters with patients in hospitals, in families, and in the community.

The Theme of Self-Effacement. Every human being has worth, but not all share that perception to the same degree. Evolving from past hurts and imagined slights, which are indelibly pressed upon one's memory and recalled with today's innuendos and oversights, the instinct for interpersonal survival is achieved through a publicly communicated defense — self-effacement. It is not a mechanism for erasing those indelible marks left in one's memory. It is both verbal and nonverbal testimony, which supports behavioral attempts by one person to reduce his significance, dismiss his efforts, or shrink from the self-assertion necessary to the maintenance of his ego-identity.

The expression of these feelings and attitudes is proportional to the intrapsychic pain of past experiences. In time, such expressions can become a behavioral pattern in everyday communication. When an ego-threat is serious enough to produce higher levels of anxiety, self-effacement emerges, with stronger behavioral expressiveness.

What forms of communication can such feelings and attitudes assume? Verbally, as an example, they can appear to contradict compliments for a particular effort, such as in "Thank you, but anyone could have done it." In this statement, the person who received the recognition or compliment subtly disperses his efforts among other people, thereby reducing or dismissing the real effort he invested in the task. In addition, the qualifying aspect of the word *but* suggests discomfort in accepting recognition for one's efforts. Likewise, the statement may be more direct, such as in "Thank you, but I didn't do anything" or "It was nothing really." The focus in these examples remains upon the person for whom the compliment is intended, and the devaluation of his efforts is self-inflicted, that is, he does not hide in the group obscurity of the term *others, anyone,* or *they.*

Other forms of verbal communication may suggest apology, which may place the receiver of the communication in a position of having to give permission for something not his to give. This places the self-effacing person in a seemingly subservient, humbling, and often pathetic light. Verbal communication such as "I hope you don't mind that I did this" or "If it's not okay for me to do this, I hope you'll let me know" may suggest a self-effacing theme.

Most of us and our patients have used these types of comments at some time. This does not mean that problems exist in this area. One instance does not indicate a theme. Identification of a theme implies that the communication we have received is *prevalent* and *recurrent* during the course of our encounters with that patient.

Nonverbally, self-effacement themes may be conveyed through a person's demeanor, which includes his behavior at a particular time, and the dress, carriage, and expressions that accompany it. We should notice whether his clothes are innocuous, of bland colors, loose-fitting, out of style, or carefully selected and correct. We should make a mental note of whether he stands straight, is slightly stooped, seems ready to run, or blends into the woodwork in a group of people. Whether a patient looks hesitant or begs attention nonverbally before speaking should also be a part of assessing the presence of this theme. Such nonverbal conduct can corroborate his verbal expressiveness or be abrasive to it by drawing attention to his bad points in order to satisfy his need for castigation.

Many people living among us think of themselves and relate to others as if they were an insignificant embarrassment, whose persistent theme comes as self-inflicted put-downs. The underlying reasons are many; the need for reassurance, recognition, and acceptance is great. The opportunity for beneficial nursing actions depends in large measure upon our ability to recognize the prevalence of this theme.

The Theme of Poverty. As we become more in volved with the health needs of a community and the people in it, we also become aware of another, less tangible theme of communication, whose core crosses the boundaries of race, nationality, religion, and geographic location. This is the theme of poverty, which is understood by those who are a part of that milieu, but often is incomprehensible to those of us not within the boundaries of its experience.

The experience of poverty does not refer to the lack of financial security alone; it refers to the paucity of life experiences, which are necessary to personal enrichment, and which have impact and meaning that can be shared with a variety of people. In the sense that people are left wanting in so many areas, we are referring to them as "the psychological poor." They represent people "who manage to eat enough to keep going but who suffer as keenly as those below them on the economic ladder because they have so little hope of ever enjoying what the rest of society routinely enjoys" [3]. Today's psychologically poor are different from their counterparts in the thirties, the difference being "a feeling of *temporary* exclusion from the good things of one's society and deprivation as a *permanent, even hereditary* way of life . . . It is the children and the grandchildren of these same long sufferers who are the hardcore problems today" [4].

Anthropologist Oscar Lewis describes the efforts of people within the culture of poverty as "local spontaneous attempts to meet needs not served in the case of the poor by institutions and agencies of the larger society, because the poor are not eligible for such service, cannot afford it or are ignorant or suspicious . . . it is both an adaptation and a reaction of the poor to their marginal position in a class-stratified, highly individuated, capitalistic society. It represents an effort to cope with feelings of hopelessness and despair that arise from the . . . improbability of achieving success in terms of the prevailing values and goals" [5].

As we become more aware of and are exposed to more of the realities of poverty that beg to be recognized within our communities, we are struck not only by the severity of the problem, but also by the realization that we are not as well equipped as we may think we are to deal with that problem. Our frames of reference, our own life styles and life space, even our communication patterns reflect the programming of our middle to upper class value systems. The point at which we would begin to help is often based upon what we consider to be the basic problem based on our value systems. It is difficult for us to understand that psychic inertia is the root of the problem. The task is not simply a matter of providing services, but of helping an individual or family find the motivational energy required to get to them so that they may be used. We cannot realistically expect an individual whose life has been filled with continual deprivation to suddenly be motivated to find the behaviors and energy necessary to fill his role in society vigorously.

The psychologically poor do communicate, but in a way that is foreign to our own ritualistic methods of communication. We often make no attempt to find whether there is some common basis for understanding through our present communication practices. More important, we are often unwilling to take the first step in that direction.

It is to our standards that the psychologically poor must submit, and upon which they are evaluated. We meet them every day in the hospital. They are our sources of frustration, our bones of contention, our source of stereotype reinforcement, and one of our greatest challenges. They may be the patient who cannot translate or remember specific instructions from day to day, even with our help, or the nursing student from a similar background who cannot describe his observations or write them. There are any number of examples. As we listen, it becomes all too apparent that there are great gaps of information, without which understanding seems unlikely. It is reminiscent of trying to plug a leak in a dike with our finger — just as soon as we do, another leak appears that requires the same treatment. No matter how hard we try, we cannot stop the water from escaping, and we soon run out of fingers to use.

Listening can also reveal a patient's difficulty in describing his needs, problems, and concerns. We must consider whether it stems from insufficient education, the pressure to perform well, or a paucity of certain life experiences. For example, a young female patient, 23 years of age, had great difficulty describing what she saw outside her hospital window. Though she finally was able to do so, it was not without a struggle for words and resulted in a very simple description, without details relative to the clothes people were wearing, the activity on the street, or the colors she saw. She may not have this problem when she is among her friends and in her own neighborhood, because she probably would not feel pressed for information.

Sometimes these people express an extraordinary candor in settings where such candor is not usually expressed. As an example, a young black nurse's aide approached her head nurse (who was white) during a Christmas party for the nursing staff. She said, "I think your uniforms look great on you, but in your regular clothes, you look fat." Such candor can be startling and can leave people at a loss for words. In all likelihood, our first temptation would be to consider such a person rude, or someone who comes on strong. Neither of these may apply. Such candor may be typical of that person's background in which private communication (in the sense that it is direct and not masked with politeness or the appropriateness to which we are accustomed) is not only socially acceptable, but also expected. Taking that factor into consideration, it would be a mistake to think of someone as rude, unless we could assess whether a remark was made deliberately to harm someone.

A nonverbal aspect of this theme that may misguide us in our attempts to listen carefully is the selectivity we use in assuming that the stylishness or lack of it in a person's dress indicates everything about his background and ability to relate to others. Thus, we are unprepared to relate with ease when we attempt to assess needs through listening and interviewing. Concerning ourselves with external signals of this kind often reminds us all too pointedly how entrenched we are in our own ethnocentricity. The psychologically poor do not necessarily look poor with respect to their clothing, talk poor, or act poor by adopting the submissive attitudes, shuffling gaits, and mumbling responses we conveniently associate with being poor.

These people do communicate behavior, which tells us eloquently and precisely about the theme of poverty. It may be a communication style rich in description and candor, one that is presented without guile and that pricks us with the barbs of reality that can only be conveyed by the people who have experienced it. The communication theme is before us, but its motifs will continue to elude us if we continue to use old ways of listening in response to new ideas.

The Theme of "ME". Unlike the theme of self-effacement, in which one tends to reduce or minimize his ego-identity, the theme of "ME" is an open declaration of one's existence. At the emotional core of both are people who are unsure of themselves. Their need to feel secure should be anticipated before their communication behavior either minimizes that need or exaggerates it. In both themes, people tend to place interpersonal barriers between themselves and others through their behavior.

The theme of "ME" is often expressed in the first person, in terms of one's actions or thoughts, which are usually direct and obvious because of *recurrent* usage. The prevalence of phrases such as *I* did, *I* think, *I* feel, *I* want, *I* told, and *I* said suggests the importance of the interpersonal *I* to the speaker.

In the hospital situation, this type of person unfortunately has been labeled "the demanding patient." He draws us into his circle of interaction by demanding favors and tasks that will ensure his ego-comfort. The demand (which really is a frightened plea) forces us to focus our attention to his plight and in so doing forces us to concentrate on the *task* and not the person. The task is often done despite the person, or as if the person were nonexistent. The endless circle of this theme is that in sensing the antagonism and, therefore, the ego-threat, the patient meets it with further demands for attention. The exasperation and multiplicity of these demands completely overshadow the real and underlying theme — the uncertainty of the "me" that no one really knows.

The theme of "ME" may be introduced even though the subject matter does not appropriately elicit that kind of communication. This is another cue for which we should listen, because we should be asking ourselves what may have prompted such behavior in the first place.

As nurses, we are not immune to use of this theme ourselves. Often new experiences and new people present enough of a threat to prompt behaviors that emphasize the professional "ME"; it both summons the attention of others and controls it during uncertain moments of an interaction. Listen to the following nurse as she encounters a patient:

> *Nurse:* Well, I was standing over here asking myself whether or not I should wake you.
>
> *Patient:* I don't want to talk. [He curls up and closes his eyes.]
>
> *Nurse:* I really feel you owe it to both yourself and me to do more than just pretending to sleep when I am here.
>
> *Patient:* I don't want to talk to you. You're a pretty thing, but there is no point.
>
> *Nurse:* I don't think you need to try to make me uncomfortable either. [I felt in control of myself, and therefore the situation did not seem personally threatening.]
>
> *Patient:* I don't particularly like you. You are not the best student nurse I've talked to.
>
> *Nurse:* I really don't see why you feel you need to embarrass me. I'm here to talk about you, with you. That's what I'm interested in and that's what I'm here for, so I suggest we begin.

Listening to ourselves, as well as to our patients, is an important element of a helping relationship, for we may find that we emphasize the "ME" theme of our communication more than our patients do. Since a helping relationship is one in which the patients' needs predominate, we can defeat our objectives if we express our "ME" theme too often. We may lapse into it in beginning attempts to establish a helping relationship because our anxieties are high and our role insecure. As we learn to effectively cope with both, the patient's themes and his needs are more easily detected.

The Theme of Wellness. Another theme for which we are unaccustomed to listening is that of wellness. We have become aware of the problems that indicate deviations from health, but components suggestive of health are often missed. In the process, we miss cues that are important in the assessment of a patient's health status and that would give us greater insight into his well-being.

Before we can do this, we must become much more familiar with the standards that can function to guide our listening abilities. The guidelines contained in various physical and psychosocial need categories, developmental tasks, life crises, and concepts of positive mental health, to name a few, equip us for the development of listening pursuant to the theme of wellness.

In the activity of listening, we seek information that is pertinent to the theme. For this, inquiries into what brought a patient to the hospital, for example, may help us begin to identify his areas of wellness. Similarly, by eliciting descriptions of a time in which he considered himself well or of what he might do when his illness subsides, we identify what he sees as his level of wellness. By comparing it to his need, problem, or illness, we can assess whether the theme of wellness is within realistic proportions.

The discomfort we experience in listening for this theme is not only that of disappointment because we have not discovered a problem, but also that of not knowing what to do once we have identified it. Listening for evidence that substantiates themes of wellness allows us to assess not only the patient's perception of his level of wellness, but also the manner in which he maintains it and the factors of everyday living with which he must cope in order to do so. In addition, we can listen to detect the reality of his perceptions of wellness. For instance, does a patient still entertain perceptions of wellness that exclude *any* problem, *any* degree of infirmity, or *any* disruption of his life style despite the fact that an illness is being experienced? Does he measure wellness according to the things he is able to achieve and the attitudes he is able to maintain even in the face of problems or illness? Even though the theme of wellness is expressed positively and indicates a good mental outlook, it is a theme that still needs to be assessed through listening.

The Theme of Loneliness. No theme is as poignantly expressed as is loneliness. It can be pervasive or explicit; the ache in a life style or the outcry of a single experience. It is a concept against which we all defend with a maze of words and behaviors.

We are all lonely people in the sense that at varying times in our lives we have experienced a moment or two of isolation — of apartness — in which others could not reach us and to whom we could not extend ourselves. The void — the emptiness — a kind of vacuum, which envelopes and consumes the interpersonal meaning we receive from others — has been written about often, and no more notably expressed than in the words of T. S. Eliot:

> We are the hollow men
> We are the stuffed men
> Leaning together
> Headpiece filled with straw. Alas!
> . . . .
>   Shape without form, shade without colour
> Paralysed force, gesture without motion [6].*

Psychologists, psychiatrists, and sociologists have attempted to give it definition, determine its etiology, and prescribe remedies, but it remains the solitary experience of the person who lives in its shadows. No one feeling was ever so suited for the sincere compassion of a listener — one who would try to experience another's perceptual void, however momentary.

*From "The Hollow Men" in *The Complete Poems and Plays 1909–1950* by T. S. Eliot. Copyright © 1962, by permission of Harcourt Brace Jovanovich, and Faber and Faber Ltd.

Feeling lonely and acknowledging it openly are two different things, both of which are not encouraged in our busy, active society. We take pride in our activity, our popularity, and the variety of our diversions. Like ancient, rusted armor, our pride protects our needs from discovery by others, but it is unable to defend us from the compassionate listener who senses what remains hidden. Such was the case of the following nurse, who describes her interaction with a patient:

> [Annie approached me in the corridor yesterday as I was leaving the day-room.]
> *Patient:* What's your name? [Her hand was extended.]
> *Nurse:* Margaret Hall. You remember me, don't you?
> [I took her hand and held it tightly. She mumbled a series of words and had a faraway look in her eyes. I felt so badly for her because she appeared so pathetic. I felt she was trying to tell me something, but I did not understand what it was.] Annie, I don't understand. [She continued mumbling. I heard the words *love* and *never*.] Annie, listen to me. [She became silent.] What does *never* mean to you?
> *Patient:* Never, never, never leave me alone.
> *Nurse:* Annie, we're here. We won't leave you alone. Is that what you mean? [Silence — a small smile appeared and then a searching look in her eyes. I felt I must take this a step farther since I thought she was trying to get something from me.] Annie, are you afraid?
> *Patient:* Yes. [Silence. She was still holding my hand tightly. I remained silent and thoughtful.] You've been there too haven't you?
> *Nurse:* No, Annie. I have been lonely, but I don't think it compares to what you are feeling. [Tears came to her eyes; she smiled a small smile. Tears also came to my eyes as I looked directly into hers. I squeezed her hand and felt she was accepting what I had said.]
> This experience for me has been perhaps the most moving one since I've been here. It is the first time a patient has really let me "in." I wanted to share this experience with the class, but it is even hard for me to express on paper something so deep. If this never happens again, I have experienced it once, and I feel I know what true loneliness means to one patient. I'm not sure what this interaction accomplished, but by sharing her feelings with me, Annie let me see what it is possible for me as a nurse to do, and I thank her for that.

When this need is intruded upon by illness or some insidious, relentless anxiety, protective instincts surge forward to protect us against feelings of isolation or painful solitude. In the aged, it may have the look of apathy and the sound of yesterday. Bygone days once again are filled with people and purpose, and these memories are infinitely better than the starkness of today. In people of all ages, it may result in greater efforts to discover diversions, thereby minimizing the time they are alone with themselves and their thoughts. Loneliness implies a threat that one may become a nonbeing, which creates anxiety and the pain and discomfort we associate with loneliness. The distress is unrelieved if there is no one to whom we can turn or no one who will follow in pursuit.

Listening can become an interpersonal pursuit, one dependent upon various cues expressed by our patients and our ability to understand them. Cues that should alert us are indecisiveness or ambivalence about being with other people, lack of enthusiasm for the company of others, and insistence that one is happy and leading a full life when in reality it has become more constricted. Careful attention must be devoted to a person's description of his feeling, because he may be describing lonesomeness (i.e., that he misses a certain person and wishes to be in their company), which differs considerably. Elements of loneliness may be expressed in statements such as: "I don't care"; "I have no one who cares"; "I can't seem to talk to people"; and as a patient once said, "Even God has deserted me."

Conversely, behaviors that express defiance, a chip-on-the-shoulder attitude, insistence on independence ("I can do it myself"), or withdrawal from close interpersonal relationships by a self-proclaimed loner, may suggest loneliness. By reaching across these expressive barriers and compassionately grasping our patients with the gentle insistence of the willing listener, we can begin to lessen the void, which has existed too long.

The Theme of Loss. For most of us, death is the ultimate loss — the final experience made irretrievable through the cessation of life processes. As a part of that final experience and to expiate the funereal rites of passage, we progress through the various stages of grief and mourning as if saluting the person who has died.

Themes of loss are for the living to experience. They include far more than death and extend into both the tangible and the intangible elements of our lives. Surrounded as we often are in the hospital with the intimacy of death and the problems faced by the dying, we tend to overlook other losses which are keenly felt and of significance to the people experiencing them. They can include the loss of health, home, a pet, pride, a job, and even memoirs, as one elderly lady related to her nurse:

> You know, I have twenty-six grandchildren and six great-grandchildren. I wanted to leave them with some recollections of what life was like when I was young and what their parents were like at a young age. I worked on those memoirs for two years and wrote them by hand, because typewriters and I just don't get along. When they were ready, I took them to my son's place to have him go over them. I laid them down on a table for a while and by accident they were thrown into the fireplace. Whosh — gone up in smoke. Two years of work gone — just like that. Well, I really felt its loss. It was as if an old friend had died. I grieved as if one *had* died. I'll try to do it again, but it won't be the same.

She was expressing not only the loss of her memoirs but also the loss of emotional energy and time in writing them.

Similarly, loss of youth is a familiar theme in the elderly, because they are unable to understand what has happened to make them suddenly be considered old. The inability to understand the process of one's own aging can precipitate a crisis, which psychologist Robert Kastenbaum calls the crisis of explanation [7]. Becoming old is perceived as an *unexpected* event and, therefore, it cannot be explained with emotional or intellectual comfort. Some people need an explanation of this unexpected misfortune (which is their perception of it), and it must be both plausible and comfortable to accept.

The loss of one's youth is very painful and very difficult to explain, not only to one's self, but also to others. How does one go about explaining with believable credibility that he is not what he used to be? Although the crisis may be the explanation (an attempt to reconcile what once was with what now is), the theme is loss. For some it takes the form of a complaint: "Who wants to associate with all *those* old people?"; "Old people do nothing and only talk about *their* aches and pains"; or "I'm not ready for a senior center yet — that's for old people with nothing better to do." For others, physical manifestations of aging are focused on the social acceptability of physiological symptoms: "I was quite active before this pain in my back started. Guess it's a sign of old age, but if it were gone, I'd really show you what I could do."

Other people cling tenaciously to their memory of youth by wearing apparel and makeup more suited to an eighteen-year-old than a person of sixty or seventy. Looking youthful is not the problem within the context of this theme, instead, it is altering one's appearance in order to be what one is not in terms of age. The aging movie queen of the film "Sunset Boulevard," for example, is depicted as an elaborately clothed and made-up woman, desperately trying to recapture past glories and past roles, which are better suited for younger actresses.

These types of verbal and nonverbal behaviors, which may result in a crisis if a person cannot come to an emotional and intellectual reconciliation regarding his aging, are used to protect oneself from the perceived loss of ego-integrity. To a certain degree, it is an inherent threat in anything that someone feels is personally significant. As these themes are expressed, listening becomes a means of lending ego until a patient finds resources within himself to adequately function again.

Humor as a Theme. Among the various means we use to relieve our tensions and anxieties, humor is the most welcomed and pleasurable. It is our way of enjoying the imperfect in an open, socially acceptable way. Its spontaniety and ability to provide a common denominator among people of diverse backgrounds are highly valued in contemporary society. When that world is reduced to the confines of a hospital or to a community in which people are troubled, its importance becomes paramount. Though the themes often are difficult to discern, we must discover what humor conveys if we are to be more effective in dealing with the problems facing our patients.

Humor, as Robinson points out, serves several functions, among them the relief of anxiety, the expression of hostility, and the perpetuation of denial behavior [8]. The *way* these are expressed and the type of humor used to express them are the things for which we need to listen during our contacts with patients.

Ridicule, for example, is a type of humor that often emerges during some patients' communication, and it can be directed against oneself or others. In a general sense, to ridicule is to disapprove or hold in contempt. It suggests a conscious attempt to attack a person or object in such a way that it becomes absurd or preposterous in the eyes of others. Although there are a variety of ways this form of humor can be communicated, it is usually verbal. In the case of self-ridicule, the verbal attack is self-directed and focuses on those events that directly involve the individual.

Comediennes, such as Phyllis Diller and Joan Rivers, exemplify comic styles used successfully to draw audience attention to themselves, not as they *are*, but as they depict themselves to be — a larger-than-life caricature, whose daily problems and encounters are ludicrous in the eyes of others. In the case of Miss Diller, this is accentuated by her dress and the use of her laughter. The success of comedian Don Rickles, on the other hand, is based upon the calculated insult, which he uses to flaunt the apparent imperfections of others in public. Any element of truth in the insult is magnified, so that it appears absurd to those listening. The apparent incongruency between fact and fiction may well be the spark that touches off the laughter of the audience. In some vicarious way, our tensions are momentarily relieved as we enjoy some hidden wish fulfillment by engaging in this form of humor.

Ridicule in patients' behavior patterns, however, may indicate more significant feelings, problems, or perceptions. A patient may need to direct ridicule toward himself in an attempt to evoke a response from others that will not only refute the ridicule, but also reassure him of his self-worth. This may be part of a lifelong feeling of insecurity, inadequacy, or worthlessness, which is reactivated in times of stress or anxiety and released through humorous channels. In assuming the role of the clown, for example, a person may be expressing his needs for attention and his feeling that this is the only way to gain acceptance from his peers.

At these moments, the need for acceptance may overshadow his sensitivity for the feelings of others, and his remarks may become more caustic, pointed, and blatant. The vulnerability of others becomes his target, though this is the same thing which he defends himself. By projection, he now attacks the very thing he finds unacceptable in himself. An example of this might be a patient pointing to an obese person and saying: "Look at him; I bet he does all his shopping at the Army Surplus Store — tent dept!" If the patient is obese, he may indulge in self-ridicule by a variation of the remark: "My clothes are all made by Omar, my local tent maker; he does wonders with burlap and canvas!"

Illnesses that alter a person's body image or self-image may also precipitate self-ridicule. If he is threatened by a potential or real loss but cannot express his feelings directly, humor becomes the vehicle by which they are "acceptably" released. His anger, frustration, and anxiety are aimed at himself through self-ridicule; he "beats others to the punch" by putting into a humorous context the thoughts and perceptions he imagines others have about his plight. Patients who have suffered the loss of a body part through amputation or who have been disfigured or crippled may resort to this type of humor.

Because of the generally infectious nature of humor, it is hard not to respond by giving an inordinate amount of reassurance. We cannot react by scolding, because that does not bolster a patient's self-concept. It is harder yet to resist the temptation to play along and continue the humorous exchange. It is essential that we first recognize that such a pattern exists and then determine which communication approaches will not reinforce a patient's need to ridicule himself or others.

Sarcasm is another form of humor we encounter with patients. It has a lacerating effect upon those to whom it is directed, and its roots are nurtured by an active, contemptuous dislike of someone. It is most often expressed verbally, and unlike self-ridiculing humor, it often expresses the opposite of what is actually stated. Most of us are more likely to respond to the tone of voice, the attitudes, the expressions, and the underlying feelings that are being conveyed than to the literal remark. The following exchange is an example:

> *First person:* What a nice outfit you have on today.
> *Second person:* Why thank you. You care.

The translation of the response depends on *how* it is conveyed and *where* the emphasis is placed.

The goal of sarcastic humor, regardless of the witty and often clever ways it is expressed, is to belittle or demean others. To a certain extent, it is an acceptable form of humor at social gatherings if it does not get out of hand. It is a shaft of anger in the guise of humor, which is delivered with stiletto accuracy. When it strikes, it cuts deeply, and we respond to it with the instinctive behavior we use to defend ourselves. This type of exchange can raise anxiety levels high enough so that it inspires more sarcasm, not less.

It is often difficult to determine if sarcasm is a deliberate act, the product of momentary stress or anger, or integral to a person's behavior. It can be as much of a surprise for a person to be told he is being sarcastic as it is for another person to find that he is the target. In the effort to belittle, the person who uses sarcasm succeeds in putting down his antagonist and momentarily achieves satisfaction and the superiority he may need to feel in that situation. The adage that "the best defense is a good offense" aptly describes the use of such humor.

For a patient this can be a successful avoidance maneuver, because when he is engaged in sarcastic humor, he is temporarily evading reality or a situation with which he must learn to deal. Frequent use of this mechanism may indicate his unreadiness to deal with the anger his anxieties may have generated. Unable to discharge his feelings directly, he must find a way to do so that is socially acceptable and economic to his threatened ego. Control, therefore, is essential to execute the sarcasm and to preserve his self-concept and ego-integrity. Loss of control, which is often synonymous with succumbing to anger or hostility, is perceived as a dreadful alternative for a patient whose ego cannot tolerate more stress than it can constructively accommodate.

With patients who continue to use sarcastic humor as a means of dealing with their anger, hostility, and anxiety, it is especially important *not* to respond in kind. Patients who find it difficult to trust others and who already perceive us as disapproving figures of authority may interpret such responses as attacks. Their high anxiety levels do not permit them to perceive them as anything else.

The poignant aspect of such humor is that, despite the wit and cleverness, it succeeds in driving people away, and this is not what an insecure, anxious patient wants or needs. If we respond in kind and retreat from further interactions with him, we only reinforce the things that do not need to be reinforced.

As difficult and uncomfortable as it may be for us to be the recipient of such humor, we must learn to be as objective about it as possible. We must keep in mind that such patients have difficulty expressing their anger fully and directly. They desperately need the security of a trusting relationship that can help them explore more constructive means of releasing their feelings. By commenting quietly and calmly about the emotions they are expressing, rather than taking personal offense with *how* they are expressing themselves, we may, with a consistent approach, be much more supportive.

Ethnic jokes also merit comment, because they play a part in determining the extent of a person's stereotypes and prejudices. In an ethnic joke, some characteristics that the teller feels best represent that particular ethnic group are singled out. For example:

> There was a mining accident in Great Britain in which six men were trapped — two Englishmen, two Welshmen, and two Scotsmen. When a reporter asked a bystander what he thought the men were doing while they were waiting to be rescued, he replied, "The Englishmen are taking tea, the Welshmen have started a quartet, and the Scotsmen are taking up a collection for the widows and orphans."

Question: How many Pollacks does it take to put in a new light bulb?
Answer: Five. One to hold the bulb and four to turn the ladder.

Ethnic jokes are not as openly or playfully accepted now as they were in the past. In some areas, they are not humorous, especially to people of the same ethnic group. The issue of ethnic identity is being raised by people who take exception to jokes in which their nationality or race is ridiculed. The standard ethnic themes of these jokes, such as Pollacks are dumb and dirty, Italians are gangsters, Germans have a fetish for order, and Jewish mothers smother their kids in chicken soup, fail to amuse people in these groups. Granted, not every person within that group may respond adversely, but it may be prudent not to assume that everyone thinks such jokes are funny.

A patient who continually tells stories or jokes of this kind may be revealing a difficulty in accepting people of other races, nationalities, or religions. Prejudices based on faulty stereotypes become telescoped into an ethnic joke with a discernible "edge" to it. It gains acceptance through laughter, and the teller finds a new outlet for his prejudices. In groups of patients, or in ward situations, an "Archie Bunker" type of joker can raise the hackles of the most sanguine of them. We must listen for the *derogating* quality of the joke, because not all ethnic jokes have it.

Themes resulting from these and other expressions of humor need assessment, based on the consistency of use, the level of anxiety being experienced, its relationship to the problem or situation, and its effect upon the interpersonal relationships of the patients using it. Listening to the themes in humor, therefore means hearing more than the sound of laughter.

NOTES

1. Kemp, C. Gratton. *Perspectives on the Group Process,* p. 234.
2. Barnlund, Dean. *Interpersonal Communication: Survey and Studies,* pp. 569—575.
3. Bordiner, Robert. Poverty is a Tougher Problem than Ever, p. 76.
4. Ibid., pp. 78—79.
5. Lewis, Oscar. The Culture of Poverty, p. 5.
6. Eliot, T. S. *The Complete Poems and Plays 1909—1950,* p. 56.
7. Kastenbaum, Robert. *New Thoughts for Old Age,* pp. 316—319.
8. Robinson, Viola. Humor, pp. 133—134.

(Bibliography appears at the end of Chapter 13, pp. 216—217.)

12

Touch, Taste, and Smell

WHEN A PERSON communicates, he uses various communication symbols
to translate some perception or thought in such a way that it can be shared with
another person. In the process of translation, that event is changed; it becomes
something altogether different from the original internally experienced event.
This is not unexpected, since "most of our present day failures . . . can be traced
either to misunderstandings of the role symbols play in inter-human communication or to inadequacies in the way we create, transfer and perceive symbols" [1].

TOUCH

The act of touching is nonverbal communication. When we touch a person,
the pressure on the skin is an external event that stimulates responses within
that person's nervous system. The way touch is conveyed and the meaning
derived from it need to be described.

Touch is like a two-edged sword in communication. On the one side, it has
cultural determinants steeped in traditions and strict and forbidding social
taboos; on the other, it has an important reaching-out function that is needed
(but not fully understood) within nurse—patient relationships. Either edge of
this sword can leave its own mark, but they are interdependent, in that each
side needs the other if both are to be used smoothly.

Many culturally determined responses to touch are universal. Everyone
understands a pat on the back, a slap on the cheek, a handshake, or a tap on
the shoulder. This commonality of understanding is absent with many other
acts of touch, and they are misperceived as they are translated from our internal
experiences (i.e., our perceptions) into physical acts.

The origin of these misconceptions is in our traditions and taboos. Primitive in origin, touch was a precursor of speech and later evolved into communication symbols, which were associated with roles and events, such as healing, magic, war, and authority. As civilization became more sophisticated, its codes, manners, and mores became more intricate and its social taboos more pronounced. Touch became a part of that complex system of taboos, which often necessitated an equally intricate system of social enforcement. By employing governesses, nannies, or chaperones, families assured themselves that social proprieties were maintained. Spatial distance was used to reduce the temptation of touch, especially among young ladies and gentlemen of courtship age. All these types of social enforcement (and many more) lent substance to our perceptions of touch as both a temptation and a threat in interpersonal communication.

The perception of touch as a temptation, in the pleasurable sense, originates in the mother—child relationship. Physical contact within this very close spatial proximity fosters love, oral gratification, and closeness. These acts help that infant associate the sensation of physical contact with that of pleasure. Awareness of reality is developed as an infant comes into contact with its mother, and it is broadened with each caress, manipulation, and fondling experience. Developmentally, the consistency and congruency with which touch is used have far-reaching implications later in life.

Touch is perceived as a threat during early development generally through the withholding of physical contact. Its absence, even for a short time, provokes anxiety in an infant who may perceive it as an obstacle to tactile gratification. The prolonged withholding of physical contact during these early months of life can, as Dr. René Spitz suggests, have irreversible effects on the behavior of the infant [2]. Contact with reality is lost, and without continued experiences of physical contact with some consistent and significant person, feelings of helplessness and unreality increase. As the need for physical contact becomes more imperative, the search for sources of it becomes urgent. In other words, when the need for contact is greatest, any source is preferable to *none*. In Harry Harlow's research studies of maternal deprivation in monkeys, mothers made of wire or cloth were far more preferable than having no mother at all [3].

In the developmental process, children become aware, through subtle and instructional forms of communication, of the social taboos that govern the use of touch, and therefore learn the proprieties employed in interpersonal relationships. Touch, the primitive means of communicating that has been a source of comfort and pleasure, must now be used carefully and within the perimeters of social acceptability.

A substitution takes place in which the actual experience of physical contact is replaced with the linguistic experience of touch.

According to the psychologist Sidney Jourard:

The metaphor of "being turned on" describes the experience of physical contact. When part of your body is touched you can't ignore that part of your body. It becomes [the] figure in your perceptual field. You might say that that part of your body comes into being. [Similarly] the metaphor of "being touched" as in the expression "your plight touches me" is relevant here. There are many touch associations in our language and in our everyday experiences [4].

In this same vein, poets, writers, and lyricists give us the emotional sensations of touch through the imagery of their words. These allow us to enjoy the pleasures without the actual experience, while at the same time, they attempt to describe the sensations derived from the experience of touch. Words such as these are an attempt to describe the sensations derived from the use of touch, when in reality such words may be unnecessary. Use of touch during adult life is restricted to the amenities that have been preordained by society. The boundaries of reality so necessary during childhood now become spatially invisible, but they still separate us from others. Within this wall, touch bridges "the gulf many people develop between themselves and others, and between their 'self' and their body. To be touched is an almost infallible way of having one's attention seized and diverted from anything it was occupied with. Touching another person is the last stage in reducing distance between people" [5].

Although touch is a crucial factor in reducing physical or interpersonal distance between two people, its potential threat is in the meaning being conveyed. Unless the communication extended through touch is mutually understood, it can pose a threat sufficient "to invite violence or panic" [6].

Nursing Considerations

Given the role and development of touch in past and contemporary societies and the potential for misinterpretation, its use in nursing poses several problems for consideration. Many nursing tasks involve touch, which is in a context generally accepted and understood by our patients. They understand its use in our nurturing role, because the communication conveyed as we hold infants and children, give backrubs, and bathe patients is well established by traditional antecedents.

In addition, using touch in nursing is closely allied to spatial distance; that is, certain uses are expected and accepted within territorial limits that might otherwise not be tolerated. For example, care of a severely ill patient or physical restraint of a restless patient requires close physical contact, and it is permitted because each member of the interaction assumes a role, in which a certain type of behavior is expected.

When someone assumes the patient role he requires more close physical contact than he ordinarily would tolerate at that same spatial proximity during health. Illness prompts regressive behavior, which is acceptable within the patient role and makes physical contact a more acceptable need. Similarly, our role as professional nurses allows us additional privileges of physical contact.

Even within the security of these roles, intrapersonal comfort may be difficult to achieve. We often find ourselves braced against the inevitability of physical contact with patients. We stiffen, flinch, or back away from gestures that suggest the possibility of being touched. Nevertheless, they are tolerated and accepted because of the specific roles assumed within the relationship.

As nursing has begun to extend beyond traditional role boundaries, accompanying role behaviors have also undergone reassessment and change. When the roles were initially extended in the area of psychiatric nursing, the ramifications of touch within the nurse—patient relationship were revealed. Because the patients' encoding and decoding abilities were already severely hampered by distortion, their interpretations of the use of touch varied widely.

The use of touch is difficult for us to assimilate to our professional role, because of our sociocultural backgrounds and our traditional concepts of nursing. Although we recognize the influence of high levels of anxiety upon a patient's perception as well as our own, and we are beginning to appreciate the influence of our sociocultural backgrounds on our attitudes toward physical contact, touching others and being touched in return still have an element of uncertainty.

Within the community, where we are not confined to the props and symbols of our role, we are often uncomfortably aware of our hesitancy to touch someone. If we are not familiar with the ways we use it or the things that influence its use, we enter interpersonal situations without the information and perceptions necessary to two-way communication. Similarly, we need to become exposed to and learn how touch is used within various ethnic cultures. Any interaction that is initiated by touch before we are ready to understand it can add strain to the exchange that follows.

In the community, and, to some extent, hospitals, nursing has become a reaching-out process in which we experiment with new roles, new ways of communicating with people, and new ways of capturing their attention. Physical contact has become an increasingly important and visible means of facilitating this process. In a sense, it is the last communication barrier between ourselves and patients and allows us to communicate in a way that is unique from other forms. As we begin to reach out and touch people, we become much more aware of how we feel in using it and, more important, how our patients react to it. This is a new and uncertain area of exploration for us, but one not without misunderstanding.

There are several considerations that we must keep in mind as we begin to use touch in our interactions with patients. The first is that whatever value touch may have in interpersonal communication, it cannot be determined by intuitive processes alone [7]. Although research is necessary to discover the standardized meanings of touch and the common ways they are expressed, the most immediate sources of information are nurse—patient interactions. Then we can assess how patients use touch and the meanings conveyed through its use. Likewise, we need to assess our level of comfort and response to patients who attempt to reach out to us. We must learn the signals patients send to tell us not to touch them because of sociocultural influences or some psychopathological reasoning by which they interpret touch as an assault or sexual threat. As in other forms of communications, patterns of touch are discernible in our patients, just as they are in us. Some people can touch others, but shy away from being touched; others are just the opposite.

The second consideration is the use of touch as "an expression of therapeutic intent" [8]. Since the meanings of touch are varied, and the gesture is significant to both ourselves and patients, our intent must be purposeful during our interactions. This is not to say that we should restrict use of touching gestures — only that this type of communication should be used discriminately to the best of our ability, it should be helpful, and its purpose should be understood by our patients.

This form of communication, like many others, involves risk. More than likely, we will be unsuccessful half of the time in our attempts to reach out and express a therapeutic intent. We must begin again and again until we become more secure and mobilize touch into a more effective channel of communication. Successes also need to be remembered. That risk — that reaching out to another person — overcomes the many choking hesitancies and embarrassments that make verbal communication difficult.

Touch surpasses the need for words when verbal ability to communicate is momentarily halted. Such moments exist for all of us in illness and in health. Touch is inherent in various roles, such as in nurse and patient or mother and child relationships. As we expand our nursing role, as we explore the patterns and potential within us and within patients, we may begin to discover additional applications of its use during helping relationships.

TASTE

In every interpersonal encounter, our ability to perceive others is based on how fully we can use all our senses. Although we rely more heavily upon sight, hearing, and touch in nursing assessments, taste and smell can also contribute to our perceptions. Like the other senses, they are taken for granted, and their potential function is often overlooked in nursing practice. Nevertheless, they provide us with sensory data upon which our impressions of patients and their families are based.

The organs of taste and smell are connected physiologically by a web of nerve receptors located near each other — adjacent to the nasal passages and along the base and surface of the tongue. The organs rely on each other and provide concurrent experiences. For example, if food is involved, the taste buds are stimulated as the aromas from it are received by the nerve receptors for the sense of smell. The sense of taste greatly depends on the sense of smell, and when this coalition is temporarily blocked or blunted, the ability to taste also is dulled.

Of the two senses, taste seems to have less impact upon communication between ourselves and patients. It does, however, add to our knowledge from a sociocultural and a socioeconomic point of view. The offering of a cup of coffee is a cultural ritual often as important as the content of the interview, because in this exchange we can discover clues to a person's social conduct, economic status, and abilities to prepare food.

The way food is used also provides clues to topics that cannot be discussed directly. The use of food as an evasive tactic, regardless of social acceptability, requires scrutiny. In some nurse—patient relationships it is one vehicle by which a transference phenomenon can occur, particularly if the ages of the participants correspond to those of a mother and daughter, or grandmother and granddaughter. The nurturing, mothering role, which was practiced for so many years with their own children is revived as grandchildren appear, but when families are separated, this role is extended to others, such as ourselves, during home visits. This is particularly common during home visits with the elderly.

We must become aware of the economic and cultural significance of food to each individual and family, particularly if their behavior suggests that food is being used as a mode of communication. This situation became apparent during a home visit between a nurse and an elderly Italian woman. Here is the student's account:

> In the earlier phases of our relationship, serving coffee and cookies was almost a routine event. Once or twice I could hear the kettle whistle as I climbed the stairs to her apartment. I felt good about it, since I knew that Mrs. P. was expecting me and was making preparations for my visit.
> When I returned after the Christmas holiday and began preparing her for the eventual end of my visits, she seemed quieter and more thoughtful. Although I did not feel this was unusual, I was surprised that our usual coffee and cookies had become more elaborate. She offered me various cheeses, salami, and fancy cookies she had purchased. Since I was well aware that she had a limited income and that what she had purchased was expensive, even by my standards, I began to feel uncomfortable about the amount of money Mrs. P. had paid for all the food. When I spoke to her of my concern, she countered that she bought it for her

lunch and wanted to share it with me. I had no recourse but to let her do so. After the visit I decided to make sure I did not come at lunchtime again in order to avoid a similar incident.

I made my next visit at 10:30 a.m., and while I was climbing the stairs, I became aware of a delicious aroma from above. I was hoping it was not what I thought, but when I opened the door I realized what wishful thinking that was! The dining room table was set, and Mrs. P. was bringing in a dish of pasta and other hot foods she had cooked for our visit and which she expected me to eat. Again, I could not refuse, and while I was eating, it suddenly occurred to me that as long as I had my mouth full, I could not discuss anything related to termination. The fact that I had also set a time limit to this visit did not help.

Needless to say, despite the fact that I insisted she not cook a meal for me on my next visit, she did. Even though we had time to talk, she would go to the kitchen frequently to check on the food. When I moved into the kitchen, I could swear she banged the pots and pans more, so she could then tell me she could not understand me because of the noise.

To make a long story short, we never did discuss termination beyond reemphasizing the date of our last visit, which, by the way, she canceled. Although I wish we could have talked more, I certainly have seen the impact on her of the topic of termination, and how she used food as a way of avoiding it. I realize she needed to do this for me — it was her way of "doing for me," but I wish I could have told her how much our visits meant to me.

The importance of sociocultural influences on dietary habits and preferences cannot be underestimated wherever nursing is practiced. These factors often are not considered in planning therapeutic diets in a hospital, but they may have an impact on patients, especially if they involve a restriction of certain types of foods or seasoning. When these diets are continued at home, they may be even harder to regulate from both a sociocultural and an economic point of view. A lack of funds often predetermines the kind of food a person eats. In these circumstances, quantity overrides quality. Translated into practical terms, a person on a very limited income may choose a meal of spaghetti, mashed potatoes and gravy, bread, and coffee because it is filling and looks like more food for the money. A meal containing meat and vegetables is prohibitive financially. In this instance, food signifies a "carbohydrate life style"; one that is more filling than nourishing, and one that is determined primarily by one's ability to pay. The implication for health teaching in this area is clear, as is the social action needed to ensure a healthful, nourishing existence for every citizen.

The sense of taste (as it concerns food) can also be put to use in other ways within our relationships with patients. For example, it can become the medium through which definite therapeutic goals are realized. It can become a sensory tool — a neutral and socially acceptable way to elicit beneficial results that cannot be obtained through other methods. When used in situations that lend themselves to such an approach, it can promote self-esteem and ego-integrity and reactivate one's previous interests and roles. The following examples may help to illustrate:

> Mrs. B., aged 86, lived alone in a residential hotel in the downtown area of the city. She was Austrian by birth and until World War II, owned and operated her own cooking school. She was a very articulate, effusive woman who enjoyed meeting people — especially younger people. Although she preferred living alone and independently, she expressed on more than one occasion her wish to have a kitchen of her own. This wish became even more pronounced as the annual bazaar at her senior center drew closer.
>
> Sensing her need to participate and receive recognition for her culinary talent, the nursing student invited Mrs. B. to her apartment so that she might bake something for the bazaar. As they worked together, Mrs. B. used the time to instruct the nursing student in the fine points of cooking and baking. Mrs. B. also used her to taste the different batters she was preparing so that the student would know how to judge a good batter, in addition to getting another opinion about a flavoring she was adding.
>
> When no cookie cutter was available, the nursing student was pleasantly surprised to see Mrs. B.'s inventiveness in finding substitutes, which included film cartridge containers, a half dollar, and caps from various size jars. Her baked goods were the first to be completely sold out and provided Mrs. B. with a source of recognition.

> Mrs. A., a tiny lady of 75, who lived alone, did not enjoy cooking for herself. As a result, her weight began to decrease gradually, despite her doctor's urging to gain weight. She began to go to a senior center once a week, where she ate a hot lunch, but this still did not provide her with enough incentive to eat more. Together with her doctor, the senior center staff, and a nursing student, plans were formulated to see if a beneficial change could be made.
>
> The nursing student began her home visits to Mrs. A. at lunch time, since Mrs. A. expressed an interest in cooking for someone. Her interest in food began to be reactivated, and together with the student, they planned menus and compared recipes. At the same time, the nursing student and the senior center staff encouraged Mrs. A. to join the Tuesday evening supper club, which involved planning and cooking a meal for other interested members. With support, she joined and became increasingly involved as time passed. With this involvement, the doctor began to see a gradual weight increase during Mrs. A.'s periodic check-ups.

The use and importance of food can provide many cues to the life style of those with whom we come in contact. In this respect, our senses cannot be developed unless we are aware of the possibilities for their use, whatever the setting.

SMELL

The olfactory organ has been described as underdeveloped and dulled in a culture in which odors are obscured by deodorants and suppressed by air fresheners. Thus sanitized, we have become unable to tolerate, much less recognize, the odors that each culture incorporates as its own. Our sense of smell provides us with olfactory clues to the invisible boundaries that make up another person's spatial territory. These clues relate various aspects of culture, personal preferences, impending trouble, and moods. If we do not pay attention to these clues, we become less aware of odors, and as this desensitization continues, we become olfactorily deprived.

Prolongation of an odor can fatigue our olfactory receptors, but they can be reactivated with a variety of odors. In the same way, though we place much value on an odor-free environment and thus are desensitized to the smells about us, we can be realerted to the odors that give credence and identity to our society. Handling new books, new clothes, and new wood, or opening food, such as a container of coffee, stimulates our olfactory receptors and gives us sensations to remember. Many individuals enjoy familiarizing themselves with new objects in this way.

Within intimate and personal distance, we can determine through our olfactory receptors the various perfumes or after-shave lotions preferred by those we encounter. These scents often communicate the presence of a person before we actually see him. In some cases, traces of perfume, for example, linger even after a person leaves a room, indicating that someone was there before we entered. These aromas become as familiar as the persons to us. Odors derived from smoking, drinking, and eating highly seasoned foods, such as garlic, onion, and curry, also are discernible within these zones. Body odor, halitosis, and odors connected with excretory functions and infectious processes can also be detected.

Fear or anxiety are also detectable through our olfactory receptors. Some patients who are diaphoretic under stress exude odors different from those evidenced through perspiration due to intense heat or work. As yet, we do not have sufficient biochemical information to substantiate this inference. Hall, however, reports in his book, *The Hidden Dimension,* several experiments that indicate the ability of rats to determine differences in odors of schizophrenic and nonschizophrenic patients [9]. The possibility that such means of detection exist could prove useful. We do know that olfaction is a highly refined sense in animals — one that is protective and basic to survival. This example may help to illustrate:

> In a conference room on a ward of a large state hospital, a nursing instructor began a discussion of the elements of a therapeutic environment. Several students remarked how surprised they were to see the interest

patients took in things such as flowers and feeding the squirrels and birds. Several comments were made about the relative safety of these interests, since they were nonhuman and made few interpersonal demands that were threatening. In order to test this trend in the discussion, the instructor received permission to bring her dog to the ward the next time the students were on the evening shift.

When the instructor brought her dog on the ward, it adjusted easily to the new situation and although it stayed very close to the instructor, it was responsive to attention from both the students and the patients. During the course of the evening, it became apparent that with specific patients the dog was not responsive and, indeed backed away from their attempts to pet it. Although the dog did not growl or appear aggressive, the fur on its back raised slightly as it made attempts to get closer to the instructor. Encouragement from her did not alter the avoidance maneuvers of the animal. The patients to whom the dog responded in this manner seemed pleasant and interested in it.

During the evening, this incident was repeated as the same patients again tried to pet the dog. Of about six patients who received this response from it, three were diagnosed as schizophrenics.

Although this one example and the small number of patients encountered are not conclusive evidence, the incident is curious, because many other patients were encountered that evening to whom the dog responded warmly.

At greater social distances, odors assume a thematic quality; they are connected less closely with specific individuals than with a group of people or the purpose of that group at the time. A hospital corridor or a large ward, for example, may have the general odor of disinfectants; a nursery may smell of formula or baby powder. The smells of Christmas, as family and relatives come together for the holidays, are familiar; the bayberry candles, pine cones, evergreens, and hot, spiced wine all take precedence over the identifiable odors of individuals. In other groups, the odor of marijuana is the olfactory theme, even though not everyone may be indulging in it. The orientation we receive from any number of situations involving groups of people in social distance may lead us to pursue additional clues that involve our other senses.

At public distance, individual and group distinctions on the basis of odors are not as evident. Instead, our sense of smell becomes refined on a cultural level, an area that requires more development and appreciation. Many people walk about the streets of their communities with a nonfunctioning sense of smell; they cannot distinguish one neighborhood from another. For example, they fail to notice the differences in the quality of the olive oil used for cooking in Spanish and Italian neighborhoods and restaurants. They do not detect the salty fragrance of the air mixed with the odors of steamed crab near fishing wharves. Cooked rice, incense, and Jasmine tea mark a Chinese neighborhood in the same way that barbecued spareribs may indicate a black neighborhood.

The odors of food are not the only scents that we discern as we familiarize ourselves with a neighborhood. The smells of musty hallways, mice, dampness, and decay are also there. In many ghetto areas, the smell of urine is prevalent in the hallways of apartment houses. Gas is a pervasive odor the moment we enter some buildings. Insect spray is another frequent odor in these areas, and one that can be dangerous if overused:

> One of the first things Miss M. noticed as she made her first home visit to Mr. C., who lived in a housing project, was the overwhelming odor of insect spray. When she entered, she found it momentarily difficult to breathe. She observed that all the windows were shut in the apartment. When she asked if she could open one, Mr. C. refused, stating that more bugs and roaches would come in, and he had enough trouble with them as it was. Although he was accustomed to the odor, he did complain of difficulty in breathing, but this did not change his mind concerning excessive use of the spray.

Often the odor of marijuana, whiskey, beer, or wine is detectable in apartment houses (and in local parks, too).

The activities and industries in a neighborhood can be perceived through our olfactory receptors. Stockyards, foundries, paper mills, coal and lumber yards, freshly cut grass, outdoor cooking, hardware stores, delicatessens, old-fashioned drug stores, breweries, print shops, and flowers give neighborhoods within a community a character all their own and are a storehouse of memories for its residents that an outsider may not be able to understand.

When we enter a neighborhood, these are the types of odors we need to recognize and appreciate, so that through them we can learn not only the neighborhood's attractive aspects, but also the negative factors, such as noise, soot, and pollutants, which need to be reduced or eliminated. When families living in older neighborhoods, ghettos, and run-down housing projects become desensitized to the odors that directly affect their health, our task becomes more apparent. We must find a way to resensitize *all* their senses and to help them learn the changes that are necessary for their well-being.

NOTES

1. Kaiser Aluminum News. *Communications,* p. 14.
2. Spitz, René A. Hospitalism. p. 53.
3. Jourard, Sidney. *Disclosing Man to Himself,* pp. 65–67.
4. Ibid., p. 65.
5. Jourard, op. cit. (note 3), p. 136.
6. Ibid., p. 137.

7. De Augustinius, Jane, Isani, Rebecca S., and Kumler, Fern R. Ward Study in the Meaning of Touch in Interpersonal Communication, p. 279.
8. Jourard, op. cit. (note 3), p. 66.
9. Hall, Edward T. *The Hidden Dimension*, p. 49.

(Bibliography appears at end of Chapter 13, pp. 216–217.)

13

Creativity: A Sense for Freedom

THERE ONCE WERE two men who lived in a village located on the Equator. One evening during dinner, both expressed a desire to go to the North Pole. They were intrigued by what they might find there and began discussing the routes they would take. To their dismay, each man proposed a different route. The first man insisted that the best and only route to take to the North Pole was to head north. Just as insistently, the second man felt that the best and only route to take was due south. So vehement was their discussion and so strong the conviction of their beliefs that they made the trip separately. One man headed north, and the other headed south, and *both did*, in the end, *reach their destination.*

Creativity is like that. Two people — each with the same goal — each reaching that goal in a different way. Who is to say which one is right or which is wrong? The goal has been reached — the point made.

Creativity comes in many forms and is lodged somewhere in each of us. It does not become just a tangible product — something we fashion from stone, sketch with paints, or write; it goes far beyond that. Creativity includes our ideas, the decisions we make, and the way we build relationships and solve problems. These are the results of our cognitive sense, that is, "the process by which we organize, interpret, and relate the information that our senses gather, [it is] the process of knowing, [of] having sorted out [incoming] data, classified them, and interpreted them in relation to prior experience[s]; [each of us then] associates them with [our] present purposes. The end product of these processes is what we call knowledge" [1]. Whatever the creative product such knowledge brings about, it cannot come about without our sensory processes.

Our senses are perceptual antennae, giving us knowledge of the world about us, and it is because of them that we become creative human beings. Creativity is not some special legacy given to a few; it is a force within us all. In many instances, it is dormant — untried and unused — because we are intimidated by the successes of others, by the fear of failure in ourselves, and by the often unfair and unrealistic comparison we make between the two. Like the biblical parable, we bury our creative talent and inhibit its growth in the stifling atmosphere of conformity.

Creativity is the sense *for* freedom — the freedom that comes from the degree of openness we use to the people, events and experiences we absorb through our senses. Though we may all strive for similar goals, such as health, a good job, and marriage, we have freedom in the *way* we express ourselves and direct our energies with respect to those goals. Its pursuit is essential to our growth as fully actualizing human beings, and as we become involved in our personal growth, we begin to accumulate the ingredients that are vital to the development of the creative force within us, including "rich experiences, trust in self, openness to data, attitudes that value change, freedom from threat, and the willingness to be and to become" [2]. These ingredients shape us into a variety of distinct personalities of whom psychologist Abraham Maslow says:

> [These people] do not neglect the unknown, or deny it, or run away from it, or try to make believe it is really known, nor do they organize, dichotomize, or rubricize it prematurely. They do not cling to the familiar, nor is their quest for the truth a catastrophic need for certainty, safety, definitions and order . . . they can be when the total objective situation calls for it, comfortably disorderly, sloppy, anarchic, chaotic, vague, doubtful, uncertain, indefinite, approximate, inexact or inaccurate (all at certain moments in science, art or life in general, quite desirable). Thus it comes about that doubt, tentativeness, uncertainty, with the consequent necessity for abeyance of decision, which for most a torture, can be for some a pleasantly stimulating challenge, a high spot in life rather than a low" [3].

Most of us, at sometime or other, have fit this description.

Knowing that we are creative is not enough, because creativity does not function in a vacuum. Being creative is trying — risking, failing, and trying again. It is knowing that each of us is different, and that difference increases our growth with each experience as it changes our attitudes, values, and perceptions. Being creative means not always accepting *because* when *why not* might stimulate different and newer ideas and perspectives. It means not being afraid of ourselves and the expression and experimentation needed to become a more actualizing person and a more fully sensitive one. Creativity is a search for the individuality in us, which is found *in* and *from* other people as we involve ourselves *for* and *with* them. Perhaps the words of this young nursing student can give us a better idea of what may be involved in such a process:

Who am I? My opening statement brings a faint smile to my lips as I recall an essay written for a high school English class. Looking back, I realize that at that point in my development, my first concern was to label my emotions. It was easier that way. If one has a name for everything, he feels that a certain element of fear is minimized. It is safer than . . . who can say? Occasionally, I was not satiated and would attempt to understand why I felt an emotion. I recall long hours in the yard absentmindedly pulling at the grass as my consciousness roamed among my experiences attempting to file them in neat categories of explanation. The usual outcome of these experiences was a feeling of hopeless frustration. It's like trying to force my mind to conceive of a finite universe and then setting forth on a journey to seek those boundaries.

The uneasy feeling was a manifestation of fear — fear that I would never be capable of that knowledge. What I wanted was a concrete answer, a description. The realization that this is an impossibility came long ago, perhaps unconsciously. However, the acceptance of this fact is a new concept to me. I do not feel that true individuality is a gift bestowed at birth. Granted, each man possesses a unique consciousness but how does he develop it? Is he content to live his life accordingly to the edicts of his society and his peers? Is his personality a conglomeration of admired associates? Are decisions made by weighing opinions of others? This man is not an individual. His consciousness is a tape recorder regurgitating what others have given him.

This is a frightening thought and one might ask the question: Am I like that? Recently I have confronted myself with this question of individuality. I began noticing similarities of speech patterns among my peers and wondered who was the originator. It upset me to learn how many characteristics of my personality are borrowed and I began to think that perhaps I was beginning a collection of tapes.

In each experience I see a trend leading inward. A close friend of mine says it seems that I do not care as much about what other people think. This probably is the best explanation. I am beginning to take the responsibility for my own existence and destiny. In order to make life decisions, I feel that I must truly know myself and give purpose to my existence. I am attempting to clarify my ideals and simultaneously to develop the inner strength to support them and the adaptability to alter them when necessary. Knowing oneself is a difficult process for it is an ideal state and the time element is a lifetime.

I feel some progress [has been made]. It is largely a process of experimentation with inevitable failures, for I am the first to live my existence and there is not a true teacher to guide me. It is strange that failure and tragedy hold the most prominent position in one's consideration. Successes do not seem as apparent. Perhaps it is because we learn more from failure and if this is so, we cannot regard the experience as failure for we have made advancement. This makes me wonder if anyone has ever really failed life [4].

We bring into nursing what the poet-philosopher Santayana calls a "second naiveté" — a sense of innocence and spontaneity tempered by an inquiring mind filled with a growing store of knowledge. That quality does not disappear because we are in nursing, and the boundaries of professional nursing are not so impenetrable that creativity cannot find a well-chiseled niche within its walls. To make that possibility a reality, we must watch for signs and influences within nursing that program us into a regimen of conformity, which stifles the freedom to learn and the openness to experience we need to grow personally and professionally.

Freedom to pursue creativity in nursing, however, does not imply freedom from the responsibility that legitimately accompanies that growth. Instead, it means that for every inspiration, every new idea or innovation:

> It also needs hard work, long training, unrelenting criticism, perfectionistic standards. In other words, succeeding upon spontaneity is the deliberate; succeeding upon total acceptance comes criticism; succeeding upon intuition comes rigorous thought; succeeding upon daring comes caution; succeeding upon fantasy and imagination comes reality testing. Now come the questions, "Is it true?", "Will it be understood by the other?", "Is its structure sound?", "Does it stand the test of logic?", "How will it do in the world?", "Can I prove it?" Now come the comparisons, the judgments, the evaluations, the cold, calculating morning-afterthoughts, the selections and the rejections [5].

Being creative, therefore, means imagination choreographed with responsibility and self-discipline.

What factors prevent us from asking these kinds of questions in the development of our creative capacities? In nursing, they may include things such as imposed restrictions, a devotion to order, rigid direction, and control; factors which discourage change, new solutions, and explorations [6]. Above all, they are situations that discourage the exchange of ideas and questions. Communication, therefore, becomes essential — the lifeblood, so to speak, upon which creativity depends for its existence, because the exchange of different perceptions and experiences gives cognitive life to our imaginations.

When we engage in such communication, we increase the opportunities for creative problem-solving, a process in which the possibility of several answers is considered rather than the usual one. "As changes occur and people become increasingly unique, each human problem is different from those of the past. To find the most effective solutions for the here and now in which we behave, we need every ounce of creative problem-solving we can muster. This requires people with courage and a hopeful outlook and who are open to their experience" [7].

Problem-solving, then, becomes a less static process as its dynamic possibilities are explored in whatever nursing situation we find ourselves. Its possibilities for creative use are just as viable within the structured boundaries of a bedside situation as within a home or community setting. If we look at it as only a device that programs us into a scientific method devoid of imagination or innovation, we will lose sight of the creative possibilities that may exist and further inhibit the boldness we wish to dare in that situation.

Though our professional interest is centered on the health and well-being of our patient, it should be equally concerned with the *process* used to determine it. It is through that process that our differences come into focus as we begin to explore, test, fail, and try again whatever alternative routes we select in reaching the goal. It is that process that plumbs whatever creativity is dormant within us. It can come only if we *believe* that our unique selves can make the difference in our nursing care, and then only if we and the significant people in our lives encourage and respect these differences. Consequently, we are better able to deal with the challenges before us in nursing practice. Otherwise, we take few risks and have still fewer opportunities to learn about ourselves "in process." Situations become a threat, and problem-solving becomes a static, programmed scientific method, in which we risk nothing and contribute little to our interactions with patients.

Daring to be different, then, makes it possible for us to do even a small thing in a great, creative way. The following example may help to illustrate this point:

> Mrs. A., a middle-aged woman, was aware that she was dying of cancer. She was in the hospital with a respiratory infection, and her discomfort was constant and not altogether relieved with pain medication. It was further aggravated by the jostling and bumping that she encountered as various nurses and aides came near her bed, bedside table, and stand.
>
> The degree of discomfort and personal anguish was not overlooked by her nurse. No matter how many comforting measures she used with Mrs. A., nothing seemed to help for any period of time. After much thought about the discomfort, the nurse did some personal brainstorming about remedies she may have missed and should try. One idea she had, which seemed too simple to have been missed, was to completely rearrange the furniture in the room in order to lessen the need for bumping the bed.
>
> She drew up some sketches of all the possible ways the furniture could be arranged in order to allow for the movement of the nursing staff and for maximal comfort to Mrs. A. She settled on one that she felt would be the best and showed it to the instructor (see Figure 17). She next took her plans to the head nurse and supervisor and explained what she wanted to try and her purpose for it. Though initially hesitant, both the head nurse and the supervisor agreed and offered the services of the orderly on the ward to help her with the move. Although the moving of furniture was not the ultimate solution in ending Mrs. A.'s pain, it did minimize one very important source of discomfort for her.

There is a growing need for the development of our creative capacities in nursing. Each year brings with it new responsibilities, new knowledge, and expanding nursing roles. The community mental health nurse, the family health practitioner, the school health practitioner, and the clinical specialist in the

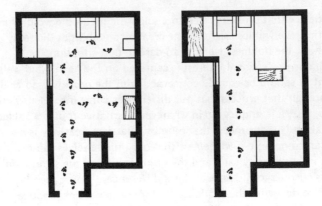

Fig. 17. Left: Floor plan of hospital room before the furniture was moved. Right: floor plan of hospital room after the furniture was moved.

hospital are a few of the new roles being assumed by a growing number of nurses. For many of these positions there are no set patterns of role behavior, no well-established rules, and traditional conduct does not seem to fit. Often these roles are not clearly defined; that is, various aspects are shared by other health professionals, or no guidelines exist to delineate their specific function.

Each nurse must discover her specific role function. For some, this sense of exploration has been stimulating and exciting, giving them opportunities to try new approaches and ideas, and sometimes to fail and later modify them. For others, the task is too much.

As these roles develop, there is a growing need for us to be exposed to as many opportunities as possible in which we can test ideas that do not necessarily conform to standard nursing procedures and approaches. The most obvious opportunity is within the nurse—patient relationship because of the potential mysteries and challenges, which can energize our latent creativity and propel it into further refinement and realization. As Moustakis explained:

> The truly human relationship is an encounter in which two persons meet simply and openly in a spirit of unity . . . It is truly bringing into activity a potential already present, or an actuality temporarily blocked or stifled. It means freeing the other person to recover *his* own nature, to express himself and to discover *his* capacities. Every act of helping another to fulfill his unique potentialities is at the same time an actualization of one's own capacity for selfgrowth . . .
> In the creative relationship, changes occur not because one person deliberately sets out to influence and alter the behavior and attitude of another person, but because it is inevitable that when individuals really meet as persons and live together in a fundamental sense, they will modify

their behavior so that it is consistent with values and ideals which lead to self-realizing ends. The creative relationship is an experience of mutual involvement, commitment and participation, a meeting of real persons. It can be studied or learned in a static and discrete sense, but it can be known only through living . . .

[In it] there is a feeling of oneness, a feeling of communion . . . It means expressing one's talents and skills immediately, spontaneously and in accordance with the unique requirements of each human situation [8].

The key to promoting the growth and health of a patient is found within the relationship. This is where we can discover and activate our creative capacities as we try to apply them to the process of fulfilling a specific need. The many patients we find sensorially deprived in the hospital because they have no familiar objects of personal significance about them beg for the creative talents we have and can put to use. This does not mean only the placement of clocks, calendars, or newspapers in a hospital room; it can mean arranging flowers with the patient's help, smelling them, reading aloud, listening to and discussing music, or engaging in some other activity that has meaning for him.

In home visits, creativity may involve helping to hem a dress, enjoying the fragrance of a garden together, or praying together. If the visits involve people who are hard of hearing or deaf, it may mean finding new or different ways of communicating so that we are understood, just as it may help us learn how the deaf communicate among themselves. For the shy or the semi-isolated person, a walk through the nearby business district may increase sensory stimuli in a novel way. Feeling new fabrics, trying on clothes or wigs, and enjoying the hustle and bustle of window shopping are experiences that can be stored in the memory and later shared with a friend or relative. An excursion to see local points of interest is a creative way to broaden a person's perceptions of a community, so that he has a more realistic idea of how it is now rather than how it may have been. By enabling these people to take snapshots, hear their voices on tape recorders, and see themselves on television (Figure 18) we are creatively providing new sensory experiences within a helping relationship and expanding the sensory perceptions of those with whom we interact.

Our creative abilities are not confined to the sensorially deprived. They can spark the exchange of feelings that may be difficult to express directly. The following examples illustrate how two nursing students used art as the medium through which they dealt with their feelings about the termination of their relationships with two healthy older people. The first example (Figure 19) illustrates how, through her drawing, a nursing student chose to tell her peer group how she felt about terminating her relationship:

Just as the ocean and the sea are boundless, so is our life contact with other human beings. Each wave, be it stormy or calm, is symbolic of our

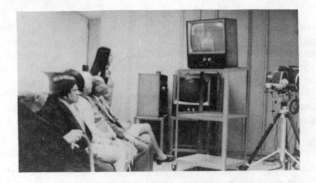

Fig. 18. Elderly citizens with nursing student viewing themselves on television in the instructional media department of the University of San Francisco.

life experiences with our fellowman. No wave ever leaves the shore without touching the million grains of sand. Be it stormy or calm, each wave supports another. As the wave recedes, a distinct line is visible just as in human relationships. The mark it leaves behind is painful and beautiful — who says that to enter a relationship would be easy?

The rock represents life. Despite being continually battered by the experiences we encounter, it endures. Through it, we continue to learn and to grow in our relationships with people.

The sand is me, and etched in the sand are the traces of every human being that has for a time touched me. Mrs. M. has touched me and given me things I can never express or thank her for. How can that be forgotten?

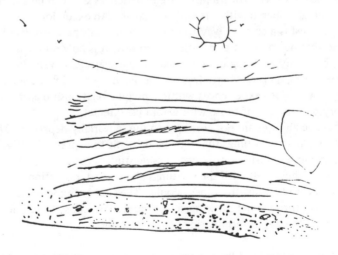

Fig. 19. Seascape depicting a nursing student's thoughts and perceptions about terminating a helping relationship.

In the next example (Figure 20) art was the medium through which one nursing student initiated and shared the termination of a relationship with an elderly woman during their last visit together. As she drew, she used her drawing as a means of conveying her feelings in the following way:

I first explored the meaning of the black blob in the center of the paper. It depicts my first conception of the aging process — darkness, loneliness, isolation, explanation, denial, death — all the crises that theoretically are possible and yet in reality are not all present in the healthy, aged individual. The darkness expressed there is the only part of my past significant to the painting in that it reveals the frame of reference from which I had moved in my relationship with a healthy older person. This point is further symbolized in every form I have drawn in the painting, which I have outlined in black. That central darkness — that first impression of aging — had been forced into the outskirts of my consciousness by Mrs. A.

The baby-blue forms not only consciously bring into focus our visit to the Tea Gardens, but also suggest, in the right form, the wings of a dove in an azure blue sky — a perception of the peace Mrs. A. has found in living — and the multitude of peace signs signifies the same victory over the crises of aging. The pink represents the effects of sensory deprivation (i.e., grotesque figures — hallucinations) by which she was not affected because she was engulfed with other people and experiences (i.e., chartreuse, orange, and blue "starve" the pink — squeeze it out of existence). Chartreuse forms represent people who use many channels to contribute to life and to dispose of life's "waste products" through coping behavior, positive relationships, and acceptance.

My optimism is related to the fact that Mrs. A. still feels the warmth of the sun's rays. If they get too hot, she is protected by characteristics

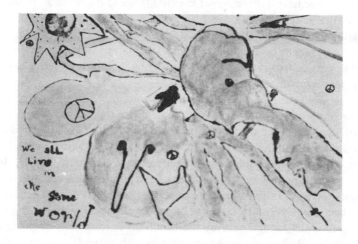

Fig. 20. A free-form drawing by a nursing student depicting various aspects of her professional relationship with an elderly woman.

of old age, namely, trust, courage, and spiritual faith in the face of decreasing physiological functioning. The sun then is life. Life sometimes gets cloudy, as does the sky, but Mrs. A. accepts the sun and clouds with equanimity; she is happy and enjoys that happiness with others. Last, I expressed a desire for someone else, such as another student, to be able to see a picture of Mrs. A.'s life and to be exposed to her as I have been.

Soon after, I gathered up my painting equipment, walked to the steps and hugged Mrs. A. goodbye. A fleeting moment . . . the time must come to say goodbye; all beautiful things must end. From them, and particularly from Mrs. A., I find myself less afraid of involvement, and through using the medium of art, have become aware of my capacity to express my feelings in a way that I hope Mrs. A. will remember as I will [9].

These are only a few of the forms creativity can assume within helping relationships. As we become more involved in new, extended professional roles within the community, we will need to explore with greater effort the creative possibilities within nursing and, more important, within ourselves. As we learn to use ourselves fully and freely in our own unique ways, we then become responsible participants in making nursing care a creative and adventurous process.

HUMOR: A NON-"SENSE"

There is another "sense," which is often overlooked in nursing practice but is used often and intuitively. It is a non-"sense", because we cannot see, touch, or smell, taste or hear it literally, yet it exists to some degree in all of us; it is, of course, the sense of humor.

Describing humor is like trying to catch rainwater in a sieve. We can witness its effects and feel its results, but it defies examination. Along with the problems, discomforts, frustrations, and joys of living, humor is a "sense" we all share, especially with patients.

There is very little humor in the dilemmas and problems of patients. Yet humor provides us with a type of adaptive behavior that allows both ourselves and patients to deal with the frustrations, contradictions, anxieties, and lunacies occurring around us in a socially acceptable way. As writer James Thurber suggests, humor is "emotional chaos remembered in tranquility" [10]. In this respect, it is the great leveler, relieving as it releases anxieties, aggressions, hurts, and angers too great or threatening to unleash directly. It offers an emotional asylum from the pain reality can inflict upon us and from feelings too overwhelming to understand. These are the functions of humor we must learn to understand in ourselves and in our encounters with patients.

Most of all, a sense of humor is a caring skill. In the gentle banter of teasing, in the shared laughter of a common frustration, and in the absurd, contradictory madnesses we may witness together, humor infectively binds us — nurse and patient — together.

Any relationship is a creative force between two people, and humor is a special type of expression that springs from it. It is elusive to describe; it may be a blend of qualities, such as observation (seeing the absurd in the pompous), boldness (voicing one's observations), or wisdom (choosing the correct moment). It may be part of the independence that permits and facilitates a flowing spontaneity between two people or of our confidence in trying something new.

Caring can come only from within; it can be expressed only by the persons involved in helping relationships. Because each relationship is unique, the humor in it is special. Humor, therefore, is a caring skill that cannot be programmed or standardized, and it should not be considered a behavior that is unbecoming to the concept of professionalism. Because humor can draw us closer to our patients, is it not a "sense" that we should cultivate? This is possible to the extent that we believe caring can be demonstrated in a variety of ways.

SUMMARY

The sensory skills of observation, listening, touch, taste, and smell enable us to transmit our thoughts and feelings to others and enable them to assimilate these messages accurately. They also are the channels through which we monitor the reactions of others. It is through our sensory equipment that our interpersonal relationships develop and are strengthened. In the process, these skills undergo continued refinement as we learn to distinguish fact from hearsay, themes from irrelevancies, and the broader dimensions we must recognize in the use of touch, taste, and smell. In addition, we must become aware of and develop two other abilities — creativity and humor — which add an important dimension to nursing practice, although they are not senses from a literal point of view.

Some principles that may guide us in using our sensory channels are the following:

1. Verification substantiates the validity and accuracy of our observations.
2. The ability to identify thematic components in a patient's communication behavior increases the effectiveness of listening as an assessment tool.
3. Listening is the primary sensory skill by which we effect therapeutic communication with our patients.
4. The therapeutic intent in the use of touch must be understood by both the nurse and the patient to be effective and helpful.
5. The responses of taste and smell to commonly experienced sensory stimuli are interdependent.
6. Creativity flourishes and requires an atmosphere of open and reciprocal communication between people who are significant to each other.

NOTES

1. Keltner, John. *Interpersonal Speech Communication: Elements and Structures*, pp. 198–199.
2. Combs, Arthur. *Perceiving, Behaving, Becoming: A New Focus for Education*, p. 144.
3. Maslow, Abraham. *Toward a Psychology of Being*, pp. 130–131.
4. Written by Catherine Nunneley, nursing student, University of San Francisco.
5. Maslow, op. cit. (note 3), pp. 134–135.
6. Combs, op. cit. (note 2), pp. 144–145.
7. Ibid., p. 149.
8. Moustakis, Clark E. *Creativity and Conformity*, pp. 136–138.
9. Drawn and written by Katherine Wacek, nursing student, University of San Francisco.
10. Bartlett, John. *Familiar Quotations*, p. 971.

BIBLIOGRAPHY (Chapters 10–13)

Barnlund, Dean. *Interpersonal Communication: Survey and Studies.* Boston: Houghton Mifflin, 1968.
Bartlett, John. *Familiar Quotations*, 13th ed. Boston: Little Brown, 1955.
Berlo, David K. *The Process of Communication.* New York: Holt, Rinehart and Winston, 1960.
Bordiner, Robert. Poverty is a Tougher Problem Than Ever. In Ned Hoopes, ed. *Who Am I?* New York: Dell, 1969.
Bullough, Bonnie, and Bullough, Vern. *Poverty, Ethnic Identity and Health Cure.* New York: Appleton-Century-Crofts, 1972.
Byers, Virginia. *Nursing Observation.* Dubuque, Iowa: William C. Brown, 1968.
Combs, Arthur, chairman. *Perceiving, Behaving, Becoming: A New Focus for Education.* Washington, D.C.: Association for Supervision and Curriculum Development, 1962.
DeAugustinius, Jane, Isani, Rebecca S., and Kumler, Fern R. Ward Study in the Meaning of Touch in Interpersonal Communication. In S. A. Burd and M. Marshall, eds. *Some Clinical Approaches in Psychiatric Nursing.* New York: Macmillan, 1964.
De Thomaso, Morita T. Touch Power and the Screen of Loneliness. *Perspectives in Psychiatric Care*, 9:112, 1971.
Eliot, T. S. *The Complete Poems and Plays 1909–1950.* New York: Harcourt, Brace and World, 1962.
Fast, Julius. *Body Language.* New York: M. Evans & Co., 1970.
Foss, Grace. Sleep, Drugs and Dreams. *American Journal of Nursing*, 12:2316, 1971.
Haggerty, Virginia C. Listening: An Experiment in Nursing. *Nursing Forum*, 10:382, 1971.
Hall, Edward T. *The Hidden Dimension.* Garden City, N.Y.: Doubleday, 1969.
Herndon, James. *The Way It Spozed to Be.* New York: Bantam Books, 1969.
Jourard, Sidney. *Disclosing Man to Himself.* Princeton, N.J.: Van Nostrand, 1968.
Kaiser Aluminum News. *Communications.* Oakland, Calif.: Kaiser Aluminum and Chemical Corp., 1965.

Kastenbaum, Robert. *New Thoughts for Old Age.* New York: Springer, 1964.

Keltner, John. *Interpersonal Speech Communication: Elements and Structures.* Belmont, Calif.: Wadsworth, 1970.

Kemp, C. Gratton. *Perspectives on the Group Process.* Boston: Houghton Mifflin, 1964.

Lewis, Garland K. *Nurse—Patient Communication.* Dubuque, Iowa: William C. Brown, 1969.

Lewis, Oscar. The Culture of Poverty. *Scientific American,* 215:4, 1966.

MacKinnon, Roger A., and Michels, Robert. *The Psychiatric Interview in Clinical Practice.* Philadelphia: Saunders, 1971.

Maslow, Abraham. *Toward a Psychology of Being.* Princeton, N.J.: Van Nostrand, 1962.

Mercer, Lianne S. Touch: Comfort or Threat? *Perspectives in Psychiatric Care,* 4:20, 1966.

Montagu, Ashley. *Touching: The Human Significance of the Skin.* New York: Harper, 1971.

Moustakis, Clark E. *Creativity and Conformity.* Princeton, N.J.: Van Nostrand, 1967.

Orlando, Ida Jean. *The Dynamic Nurse—Patient Relationship.* New York: Putnam, 1961.

Robinson, Viola. Humor. In C. Carlson, coordinator. *Behavioral Concepts and Nursing Interventions.* Philadelphia: Lippincott, 1970.

Rogers, Carl, ed. *Freedom to Learn.* Columbus, Ohio: Charles E. Merrill, 1969.

Rogers, Raymond. *Coming into Existence: The Struggle to Become an Individual.* New York: Dell, 1967.

Spitz, René A. Hospitalism. In *Psychoanalytic Study of the Child,* Vol. 1. New York: International University Press, 1945.

U.S. Department of Health, Education and Welfare. *Current Research on Sleep and Dreams.* Washington, D.C.: U.S. Government Printing Office, 1971.

Williams, Donald. Sleep and Disease. *American Journal of Nursing,* 12:2316, 1971.

Wilson, Lucille. Listening. In C. Carlson, coordinator. *Behavioral Concepts and Nursing Interventions.* Philadelphia: Lippincott, 1970.

VI

Feedback

VI

Feedback

14

Checks and Balances in Communication

NO PROCESS OR SYSTEM can work properly unless there is some mechanism by which performance is checked and malfunctions are corrected. Despite its intangibility, the communication process is not exempt from a system of checks and balances, which monitors its effectiveness. Feedback is both the mechanism and the criterion by which we can determine our effectiveness in communicating with patients.

The term *feedback* is being used with increasing frequency in the behavioral and social sciences to describe the regulatory mechanism used in determining the degree of equilibrium or homeostasis achieved in autonomous, goal-seeking systems. In inanimate systems, such as furnaces, electric blankets, and electric frying pans, the thermostat regulates the amount of heat used within the system. Providing the thermostat is functioning properly, we are assured that the amount of heat will be neither more nor less than we desire.

This regulatory mechanism also functions in animate systems, such as those within ourselves. Our respiratory system, for example, ensures a steady supply of oxygen to our bodies despite external changes. Therefore, while factors such as varying degrees of heat, cold, altitude, or humidity may readily affect our ability to breathe, the regulatory mechanisms of the respiratory system maintain a homeostatic balance between the system and the external forces challenging it.

Between ourselves and others, feedback provides a regulatory function in the system we call communication. In this process, we use feedback as a regulatory mechanism to gage the communication we receive and put into operation those modes of communication that will confirm or refute the intent of its sender.

For us it is the process of correction and of evaluation because it almost simultaneously enables us to decide which messages are understood and to initiate communication that will indicate to the sender that some are not clear.

All through life, we have absorbed a variety of communication signals and messages during our interactions with other people. In this continual process, we have learned which signals are pleasant or disagreeable, and which to avoid because of the resultant pain. These experiences teach us, or rather condition us, to behave in certain ways, and in turn determine the course of our future interactions.

The learning derived from a lifetime of feedback is crucial for each one of us, because the communication we receive from others tells us generally the kind of people we are, our value as individuals, and whether our encounters with others have been satisfying. In this respect, feedback is vital not only because we are human beings, but also because it provides us with information that can help to improve the level of our performance in achieving the goals to which we are committed.

It is essential, therefore, to maintain a system of communication that includes a feedback mechanism that is sensitive to the communication signals we receive. Without it, very little stability can be maintained within an exchange, because we no longer can count on the validity of the messages we receive. Since we communicate daily, our effectiveness depends in large part upon how readily we correct our messages and the number of feedback mechanisms or opportunities we employ. For some of us, our information and perceptual input are open and diverse, providing us with many opportunities to receive a better glimpse of ourselves through the eyes and ears of others. Other people have very few feedback mechanisms. This limits their sources of information and perceptual input, and if insufficient, can distort or inhibit what they do receive. Finally, some individuals do not realize the necessity to modify their communication because they do not realize the importance of their feedback mechanisms. They cannot be expected, therefore, to use something that for them does not exist.

TYPES OF FEEDBACK

There are several forms of feedback that offer us the kind of perceptual input we require to become more effective, including internal and external feedback. Internal feedback takes place within us. It consists of our self-perception when we think about or evaluate what we have just said or done. Regardless of the interaction or task, each triggers a self-critical evaluation of our participation in it. For example, when we try on an item of clothing we have made, our internal feedback mechanism relays back to us via the mirror information about the way the garment fits and looks on us. Likewise, when we begin to speak, we trigger a set of expectations about ourselves and about how we communicate, which is reflected in our verbal communication. When we listen to ourselves, the sound of our words and the way we speak indicate to us whether or not we have lived up to our expectations. If we have not, we must modify our verbal patterns of communication accordingly. If we have met our expectations, we experience a sense of satisfaction.

These perceptions are given additional credence through external feedback, that is, sources of perceptual input outside ourselves. Although we can hear the content and sound of our voices and like what *we* hear (internal feedback), the audience listening to what we say will determine how effective we have been (external feedback).

> We reach a high level of perception if our internal feedback information coincides with the external response. In other words, if we correct what we intend to say before we say it on the basis of what we think will be the response of the listener and the listener actually responds as we anticipated, the two systems have moved quite close together [1].

When we receive perceptual input from others that reinforces our successful efforts and helps us reaffirm our expectations, we are the recipients of positive feedback. It rewards us by returning to us many of the visible and audible signs and symbols we perceive as good. It is hard not to feel rewarded when we receive smiles, congratulations, or compliments for something we have said or done. Just the opposite is true of negative feedback — it is often perceived as a withholding of rewards and indicates that what we are doing is counterproductive to our personal effectiveness.

The reactions of the listener, therefore, are the determining factors here and indicate either a favorable (positive) or unfavorable (negative) response to what we said or did, directly influencing our communication behavior. Positive feedback is likely to promote more of the same communication behavior. Negative feedback, on the other hand, indicates that a modification is in order, which we eventually make, with time and motivation.

Still, the retention or modification of our behavior is not simply a matter of receiving positive or negative feedback. Though each of us needs *both* types, the secret is in *how* feedback is communicated to us.

Positive feedback is a rewarding source of information because it contains elements of objectivity and subjectivity. It has objectivity because as observers of the behavior and actions of others, we are not as emotionally involved as they are. Our perceptions, therefore, are more likely to be helpful and accurate and more apt to be accepted by the person to whom our feedback is directed. The subjectivity in positive feedback involves *our own* feelings about the behavior of others. Although objectivity deals with the actions or experiences of others, we internalize what we have witnessed and verbally share the effect of the event upon *our* feelings. A statement such as "I saw you looking at my answer sheet during yesterday's test, and that made me mad" indicates both the observation of an outside event and its effect upon the viewer. Objective and subjective sources of data contribute to the information needed for positive feedback.

Negative feedback, however, does not contain these elements. Instead, it consists of judgmental and interpretative sources of information. Instead of a description of an observation, for example, the behavior or event is explained; an attempt is made to introduce some motive for it. A statement such as "I saw you sitting alone at the table, but I thought you wanted to be alone" is an attempt to explain the observation of the person sitting alone at the table. A judgmental reaction to such an observation goes one step beyond. In addition to the observation and explanation the event is evaluated and an opinion given based on the evaluation. Taking the same example, we can see how this operates: "I saw you sitting alone at the table, but I thought you wanted to be alone, so I decided that if you wanted to isolate yourself like that, who am I to push myself on you." Comments such as these offer little insight into *how* communication behavior might be changed.

It is important at this point to reiterate that everyone needs both positive and negative feedback, but we should not confuse negative feedback with bad feedback. Negative feedback, constructively and specifically given about our actions or words, can help us modify them for the better. It has a bad connotation when it is poorly, vaguely, and judgmentally given. It is unlikely that we would be motivated to improve our efforts on the basis of such feedback.

PROBLEMS WITH FEEDBACK

Feedback is a helpful source of information for us, but that does not necessarily mean that we willingly receive it. We are not as open to the feedback of others as we may think we are or may want to be because of our expectations of ourselves. We entertain illusions in which we portray ourselves as we think we are or as we wish to be, and a lot of our energy is directed to preserving behaviors and actions that support our illusions. We choose, therefore, not to be receptive to feedback that conflicts with our self-image.

Because of this disparity between the perceptions of others and of ourselves, any feedback becomes synonymous with criticism, and no matter how constructively given or well-intended, it has strongly negative overtones. Feedback — an innocuous term — is equated with criticism, and on this basis is rejected.

There are many ways to demonstrate our rejection of feedback. For example, we may pay selective attention to what is being relayed back to us. This way we hear only the information that will preserve our self-illusions and avoid any that may contradict it. Suspecting the motives of the person giving feedback is another way to reject it. We try to find reasons to justify what we may feel is an unwarranted attack upon us or take exception to the meddlesome intrusion into our business. This tactic centers upon doubting the integrity of the person giving the feedback. In voicing such doubts, we persuade ourselves that the value of the feedback we receive is questionable because the person giving it may not be a credible source of information.

Related to such fault-finding is our use of rationalization, that is, giving excuses for the behavior under scrutiny. Since the real reasons for it may not be apparent, we must find some plausible excuse by which to explain it. It must sound reasonable, must not be too damaging to our egos, and must relieve some of the anxiety we may be experiencing at the time.

If none of these tactics works and our anxiety has not been sufficiently abated, a remaining alternative is to attack the person who is offering the feedback. Pointing out that person's faults and vulnerabilities can effectively (though not constructively) prevent additional feedback. If such a maneuver is pointed or severe enough, the elevated anxiety level of the other person blocks any further attempts to offer feedback in a constructive way. In fact, this type of situation can precipitate too much of the wrong kind of feedback, which is destructive and based upon judgmental and interpretative reactions. It is no wonder, then, that feedback can, from this point of view, be perceived as criticism with all its unpleasant implications.

Since these are some of the ways each of us can reject the feedback offered to us, the reason many of us are afraid to give feedback is apparent. The fear of being attacked may be reason enough for some of us, but it may be even more inhibiting if it has an accompanying threat of losing a friend or the trust of a patient, which can quickly dampen any wish to offer further feedback.

Another person's unwillingness to listen to feedback or discomfort in doing so can be perceived very early in our relationship with him. Although we may initially sense it intuitively, one overt, angry reaction will confirm our suspicions. We have several options at this point. We can offer no feedback, which implies a need for improvement; we can give only feedback that can be assessed as positive in that it supports his attempts to improve; or we can offer the kind of feedback that he *wants* to hear, irrespective of its validity. It may not be what he *needs,* but the importance of the relationship to us determines the kind of feedback that will be offered. Sometimes our needs are the motivating stimuli in giving another person what he wants, and it is easier if interpersonal squabbling is avoided when we give it to him.

Another area of difficulty is that most of us are not comfortable in sharing our perceptions or feelings with others, let alone offering feedback. In this country, open expression of one's ideas or emotions is discouraged and arouses suspicion and anxiety when offered. Our motives are often misunderstood and when coupled with lack of confidence and experience in offering feedback, we feel ill-equipped to give it to others. One reason might be that we have so few role models from which to learn appropriate feedback behavior because it is culturally discouraged. Without constructive experiences in feedback behavior, we reduce the number of opportunities not only to share our perceptions, but also to receive feedback. Our learning and the learning of others is subsequently affected.

Another barrier to effective use of feedback is the way it is communicated. Too many of our attempts are vague. The more time elapsed between the event and the feedback, the greater the likelihood of generalized statements, which indicate little that can be used for correcting specific behaviors. Immediate and specific feedback indicates to the other person that this is the way *one* person sees the situation. By generalizing, on the other hand, one presumes to speak for others, and in so doing dilutes the validity of the feedback.

Vagueness also has a dilutant effect upon feedback. When combined with lack of concreteness, such statements are difficult to correlate with a particular event or behavior. Phrases such as "That was great," "It was wonderful," or "That wasn't too hot" offer us no clues about our performance. We are left with the reactions of others, and nothing more. This forces us to plead for more information, which puts us in the awkward position of being perceived as begging or being defensive, when our only object was to ask for more specific information. Similar and recurring situations such as these can quickly dampen the desire for feedback of any kind.

We must want to learn about feedback and we must be willing not only to receive it, but also to give it so that it can be received by others who also wish to learn from it. To do this, courage is needed and a willingness to tolerate the anxiety it may arouse in us. These interpersonal factors permit us to hear with understanding and to decide and analyze *what* feedback we can use in order to modify specific behaviors.

GIVING FEEDBACK

We have repeatedly seen that, without two-way interaction, communication becomes impossible. Any attempt we make falls far short of its goal if our message is not recognized, understood, and acknowledged by another person. An offer of feedback, therefore, falls short of its goal if the other person cannot or is unwilling to receive it. The effectiveness of communication is dependent upon *how* feedback is offered and *how* it is received. Both are the lifeblood of the communication process and both require "the purposeful corrective efforts of both sender and receiver" [2].

Let us examine the various ways we can use feedback purposefully and constructively. Before we actually give feedback, we must accomplish some assessment tasks, because the data from these tasks determine what we give and how we give it. The relationship between two people (i.e., nurse and patient) has a certain sensitivity within it; our role as helping people requires that our sensitivity become an integral and viable part of that relationship if the feedback mechanism is to be used purposefully.

When we give feedback, we must be sensitive to the patient's need for it at any given time, because the demands of his problems or illness often are emotionally depleting. His energy might be at a low level and feedback may not be well tolerated. At the same time, these may be the very moments in which positive feedback may be most needed and its ego-supporting content most strengthening.

The emotional status of a patient often determines how we give feedback. It is futile, for example, to offer it to someone who is already upset or angry, because he may react negatively. His reaction to a variety of input also needs assessment, because it gives us a more complete picture of the range of his behavior patterns. A patient who is always cheerful, or always making jokes, shows us only one side of his personality. It becomes very difficult to assess how he will respond to our feedback, particularly if it deals with behaviors about which nothing can be done at the time. Such feedback deals with his personality, that is, what he is as a person, rather than the events, actions, or tasks that occur outside himself. If we are too hasty and give feedback that is evaluative (i.e., judgmental or interpretive), we must ask ourselves how such attempts help a patient. Generally, they do very little and can block his attempts toward self-improvement.

Giving and receiving feedback are influential in our relationships with patients, and they depend on factors other than assessment tasks prior to the initiation of it. The willingness to provide feedback to others, for instance, indicates a readiness to explore the procedures that will ensure its success. Although our initial attempts may seem labored, awkward, and obvious, continued practice should increase our abilities and our ease in communicating it. In addition, our willingness to give feedback is a source of encouragement to others. As we learn increasingly effective ways of giving feedback, we become role models for others who are learning to accept and use it.

Another important factor in giving feedback is the selection of the appropriate time and situation. Here, again, assessment tasks are pivotal. Timing is crucial, because feedback is most helpful when given immediately after a specific incident or behavior has occurred. In addition, waiting for any defensive feelings to subside and for the person to indicate his readiness to listen is also important to remember. Consequently, feedback may not be initiated as soon as it is possible to do so.

Included in timing is the factor of anxiety that a patient may be experiencing. Overloading him with feedback at these times may defeat its helpful intent. Regardless of our eagerness to give feedback, we must utilize the criteria that will enable us to be more effective. The point is to deliver the message in a way that is efficient, flexible, appropriate, and *heard*. Otherwise, it can precipitate reactions that cancel our efforts. For example, it may be advisable at times to understate our feedback so that we invite an inquiring response, which will involve a patient more actively in this process.

Several factors need to be considered in determining the situations appropriate to giving feedback. First, how eager are our patients to receive it? Do they ask us for specific comments about some behavior or action? What is the status of our relationship with a patient? Does it have the trust necessary for a comfortable exchange of views? Have we allowed a sufficient amount of time for feedback? If it is hurried or unsolicited, constructive attempts to provide information often are blocked. A patient receiving his first visitors after leaving the intensive care unit, for example, is not likely to be receptive to feedback that dampens his anticipation. The timing and the situation in this instance are not appropriate to the constructive aims of feedback.

Specific information is far more helpful than general information. A speech, for example, may contain several excellent points we wish to discuss with the speaker, but if all we say to him is that his speech was impressive or interesting, we are saying very little about the specific points he may need and want to know. Likewise, a nurse who confronts a patient with the statement that he is uncooperative is not helping him understand the specific behaviors or actions to which she is referring. He must, therefore, respond to the reactions of the nurse rather than to the content.

By giving feedback that is descriptive rather than evaluative (in the sense that it involves opinions or judgments), we allow a patient freedom to choose whether or not to use the information. By giving evaluative feedback, on the other hand, we offer no choice. It is thrust upon a patient often in a way that requires defensive behaviors to protect himself from the perceived threat or attack. This can only serve to block further attempts to communicate and may invite recriminations if continued. This atmosphere does not promote the trust we need to help our patients accomplish their goals. All our communication should be directed to this purpose, and the giving of feedback is an important aspect of assisting them.

RECEIVING FEEDBACK

Receiving feedback cannot be entirely separated from giving it. They occur in such rapid succession that it is difficult to ascertain where one begins and the other ends. As we send our messages, we look to the receiver to see if what we have said is understood. Just as soon as that message is begun, he begins relaying back his verbal and nonverbal signals, which indicate the degree of his understanding. Once we receive those signals, we either correct our communication on the basis of the feedback we have received or continue communicating in the same way because the feedback indicates understanding. In this way, communication is a continuous exchange between ourselves and our patients.

Two factors are important to remember in receiving feedback, both with respect to ourselves and to our patients — it must be solicited as well as wanted. If we ask for feedback, one assumes that we are interested in receiving it. It is very difficult to give feedback to someone who does not want it, feels even less need for it, and is not ready either to hear it or to receive it. We must assess the desire for feedback, because that determines how it will be utilized. For instance, the interest or wish for feedback may be minimal, and little effort is made to receive it. On the other hand, some people have an intense desire for feedback, making their requests almost impossible to satisfy. Nevertheless, the motivation for wanting information is instrumental in the delivery of it.

The more we seek feedback, the more likely we are to receive it, but the kind and quality of it depend on what we request. For example, we may inadvertently ask someone what they liked about a particular task we did. This request indicates that we prefer feedback that supports our perception. Although the receiver may wish to share several points with us, they may not be items in the same vein as the request we have made. The quality of the feedback we receive, then, may not be accurate. On the other hand, we may ask what he thought about what we did. This allows him to include in his response both positive and negative feedback, which is specific, descriptive, and timed appropriately.

By making our requests for feedback specific, by paraphrasing what we think we heard, by asking questions to help clarify the information in the original feedback, we obtain a more complete picture of behaviors that may need correction. Such information in interactions with patients increases the accuracy of perception of an event or action and allows for more objective evaluation of the information, all of which are conducive to change. The more we, as receivers, become involved in the feedback process, the less likely we are to become victims of anxiety, which makes it impossible to understand any type of feedback.

It is difficult to maintain an open, inviting, and conciliatory attitude in our requests for feedback. We cannot always be sure of what we will receive, whether we can trust the motives of those who give it, and our own responses to feedback, especially if it does not correspond to our well-protected self-image. All of these things are communicated to others and influence the degree to which they are willing to provide feedback for us. All aspects of giving and receiving feedback involve active participation of both patients and ourselves, and as we become more actively tuned in to each other, greater understanding is possible.

> The timing and amount of feedback, the positive and negative value it carries, and the interpretation (and use) made of it . . . all affect the degree of understanding achieved through communication . . . when receivers are encouraged to respond with questions, comments, corrections, or even counter-arguments, greater confidence and mutual respect are likely to result [3].

FEEDBACK AS EVALUATION

As a corrective mechanism, feedback is perhaps the most important link in the communication process. It is not only a means for self-improvement, but also a source of help to others. In our role as helping professionals, we have the means to help and the obligation to extend that help to all patients we encounter, whether in the hospital, with their families, or in the community. By providing feedback to others, we learn effective ways to be specific, constructive, and helpful. In return, we gain insight into ourselves through the feedback we receive.

Assessment enables us to plan our method of offering feedback, but evaluation of that method is just as important. The process of correction, which we and our patients, must undertake, involves reflecting, sorting, decision-making, and experimenting. It is, in fact, a process of problem-solving, but one centered on us as we receive feedback about ourselves as well as the feedback we have given. To make it a constructive process of self-correction, we must have evaluative criteria that cover all aspects of feedback. These criteria may include the following:

1. What types of questions have we asked our patients?
2. Do we individualize our approaches?
3. Which communication approaches seem to work better than others?
4. What do we remember about how we asked those questions?
5. What types of feedback have we offered?
6. In what ways did our patients respond to our attempts to give feedback?
7. What patients have given us feedback? How have we generally responded? (Are we defensive or anxious?)
8. What specific reactions to our patient's feedback seemed to emerge in us? Is there a pattern?
9. What are our conclusions regarding the feedback we have received?
10. In what ways have we begun to apply these conclusions to ourselves?
11. What changes have we made as a result of these applications?
12. What has the patient's feedback been regarding any change we have implemented?

Not all of these evaluative criteria may be helpful to us, but those that we do use, or others that are similar, can greatly assist us in making feedback a personally useful and significant tool. The questions used in evaluating our feedback abilities may help us discover the motives at the core of our communication behavior. We must seek to understand this aspect of ourselves in order that we, as mirrors, can reflect to our patients some of the answers they may be seeking to the question "Who am I?"

Our discussion has covered a variety of ideas and ways feedback can be given and received. Here is a composite of them to crystallize the discussion and bring into focus specific aids in providing our patients with feedback.

Helpful Feedback	*Principles*
1. Feedback should be specifically related to a behavior or an action of a patient.	1. Feedback that is specific gives a patient more information about the changes he may have to make.
2. Feedback should be relevant to a particular situation involving a patient.	2. The kind of situation the patient is in directly influences his ability to receive and utilize feedback willingly.
3. Feedback should be purposeful.	3. The more deliberate corrective feedback is, the more effective communication becomes.
4. Feedback should be well timed.	4. The earlier feedback can be given, the more useful it becomes in correcting specific behaviors.
5. Feedback should be descriptive and clear.	5. Clear, descriptive feedback enables a more accurate understanding of the information being given.
6. Feedback should be given only when solicited.	6. Feedback has greater meaning for a patient when he is ready and willing to listen to it; otherwise, It may increase his anxiety and reduce his ability to tolerate it.
7. Feedback should be based on the assessed needs of both nurse and patient.	7. The need and readiness to become involved in the feedback process directly influences one's ability to learn and one's willingness to correct his behavior.
8. When the feedback received is vague, clarification should be requested.	8. Feedback that is unclear blocks learning and change.
9. Feedback should be both positive and negative.	9. Patients need to know what they are doing well and what they can improve.

SUMMARY

Feedback is the last and most important link in communication. It is a process of correction and evaluation through which communication is modified. Feedback is purposeful when our efforts are directed constructively to providing both positive and negative information. From it, patients may learn not only what they must seek to improve, but also what areas of strength they should maintain. To do this, we must become aware of the problems people face when encountering feedback, and the various ways it can be provided so that it is perceived as helpful by patients. Since feedback involves two persons in interaction, our communication behavior must also be examined. The way we demonstrate our willingness and receptiveness to feedback greatly influences patients' responses to our efforts in making it a positive therapeutic experience.

NOTES

1. Keltner, John. *Interpersonal Speech-Communication; Elements and Structures,* p. 90.
2. Ibid., p. 93.
3. Barnlund, Dean. *Interpersonal Communication: Survey and Studies,* p. 232.

BIBLIOGRAPHY

Barnlund, Dean. *Interpersonal Communication: Survey and Studies.* Boston: Houghton Mifflin, 1968.
Berlo, David K. *The Process of Communication.* New York: Holt, Rinehart and Winston, 1960.
Blansfield, Michael G., and Lohrer, George F. Feedback can help You on Your Job. *Management Guidelines,* 42:9, 1963.
Davis, Anne J. The Skills of Communication. *American Journal of Nursing,* 63:66, 1963.
Keltner, John. *Interpersonal Speech-Communication: Elements and Structures.* Belmont, Calif.: Wadsworth, 1970.
Kemp, C. Gratton. *Perspectives on the Group Process.* Boston: Houghton Mifflin, 1964.
Lewis, Garland K. *Nurse—Patient Communication.* Dubuque, Iowa: William C. Brown, 1969.
Luft, Joseph. *Of Human Interaction.* Palo Alto, Calif.: National Press Books, 1969.
Maslow, Abraham. *Toward a Psychology of Being.* Princeton, N.J.: Van Nostrand, 1962.
Phillips, Gerald M. *Communication and the Small Group.* Indianapolis: Bobbs-Merrill, 1966.

Epilogue

THERE CAN BE no real end to any discussion of the communication process — only beginnings. It is dynamic; it is never static or unchanging. There are no pauses, no gaps in continuity, to interrupt what must follow; no final conclusive statements, and no programmed magical formulas designed to eliminate the ebb and flow of exchange in our interactions with patients. Despite them all, the process continues from nursing event to nurse, through messages along channels to patients, and back again to nurse — as it must, to energize, and complete the human circuitry that links nurse and patient in the mutual effort of growth and understanding. From it comes the progressive discovery of what constitutes purposeful and effective modes of communication for each of us. Through it, we discover not only what is possible to achieve but also the various communication approaches that enable us to perceive and understand the needs of the person who, for a time, is our patient and to whom we have a professional responsibility.

It is that sense of professional commitment to others that drives us on to learn the variations of approach possible in our relationships with patients. In a dynamic process, we can never be satisfied with ultimate answers and pat formulas. Our professional discontent urges us on — keeping us as away from stock formulas of communication as it does from the irrelevancies that do little to promote growth in a patient. One is stifling; the other is aimless.

Somewhere in between is the reality of a process that requires the involvement of its participants in a system of reciprocal exchange of ideas, perceptions, and feelings. It is a process of which yesterday's remedies and maxims are a part but which are not prescribed indiscriminately for tomorrow's problems and needs.

The communication process is one that we must explore with our patients, experiment in, be curious about, and ceaselessly question. It becomes a dynamic process of exchange only *after* we have been introduced to its basic principles and skills. *From that point* in time, we begin the changing, altering, discarding, and combining that make those skills part of tomorrow's process, for it will be tomorrow's patients who will have a greater need, and for whom yesterday's principles were formulated. In that tomorrow we also will be changed by a process of communication that has been integrated from the past and practiced through today's experiences. That is what *must* take place if newer, more immediate, and more effective ways of relating to patients are to be found.

No book about communication can tell anyone how to communicate — at best it can invite, suggest, advise, and caution. It is you, the reader, who must demonstrate how to communicate effectively with patients. The invitation to learn has been extended in this book; the invitation to use that learning in nursing practice is extended to you by each patient you encounter throughout your professional life.

Index